CONT~~ENTS~~

STEP
OUTSIDE
OF YOUR
CHURCH

EXPAND YOUR WORLD

David,
A great adventure in the
ministry with you.
Ala
Phil. 1:6

ALAN RABE

Step Outside of Your Church: Expand Your World © 2020 by Alan N. Rabe

Stone Crest Press
Illinois
Email: arabe@sbcglobal.net

Printed in the United States of America

Library of Congress Cataloging-in-Publication Data Rabe, Alan Norman, 1946-
        Step outside of your church / Alan N. Rabe ; foreword by Phil Tuttle ; with discussion guide.

Includes bibliographical references.
ISBN 978-0-578-78578-3

All Scripture quotations, unless otherwise indicated, are taken from the New American Standard Bible. © 1977 by The Lockman Foundation. Used by permission.

Editing by Caroline Kewney at Laser Images, Quincy, Illinois

Cover design by Scott Schaller at scottschallerdesigns.com

FOREWORD

"Seriously? A professor?" That was my first reaction in the summer of 1983 when Pastor John Treischmann of Grace Church in Normal, Illinois, introduced me to Dr. Alan Rabe.

I had returned to my hometown to serve a three-month internship at my parents' new home church. Part of fulfilling this graduation requirement before my final year at Dallas Theological Seminary was that my internship be supervised by someone besides the senior pastor who would be mentoring me.

After four years of college and three years of grad school, I was severely burned out. I longed to escape the classroom and explore the practical aspects of this life of ministry my wife, Ellen, and I were so eager to begin. Having my summer supervised by yet another academic represented everything I was hoping to escape. Whoever this Dr. Rabe was, I already knew I wasn't going to like him. He was undoubtedly the antithesis of what my arrogant 25-year-old self knew I needed!

Dr. Rabe confirmed my worst prejudices when he handed me a Summer Syllabus (an oxymoron?) at our first weekly meeting. "This guy is crazy," I thought to myself as I skimmed through the list of required reading and response papers he expected me to complete.

Sometime during that first lunch, my perspective began to change. Dr. Rabe insisted I call him Al. His explosive laughter filled the restaurant, and I could tell surrounding customers only pretended to be annoyed while secretly wishing they too could sit at the fun table.

As that summer unfolded, my new friend turned out to be exceedingly practical with a limitless passion for serving people. He gave me insightful feedback when I preached the first few sermons of my life. He went out of his way to affirm my gifts even if he stretched the truth more than a little. His wife, Linda, connected with my wife, and the four of us shared several fun adventures that were not included in my official syllabus.

It's hard to believe 37 years have passed since that memorable summer. Al and I haven't lived in close proximity since our careers took us in different directions. But whenever our paths cross, the reunion is boisterous and joy-filled. We treasure one of those rare friendships that allows us to pick up mid-sentence and build on our deep respect, shared values, and priceless memories.

I'm convinced this book offers you the same opportunity. Though it may not be as personal as our weekly one-on-one meetings, this book has the potential to enrich your career and transform your life. But you must fully engage with it. Even if you're required to read it as a textbook, open your mind to truly learn.

In these pages, you'll benefit from the hard work and integrity of Dr. Rabe's first-rate research that will hold up under the most intense academic scrutiny. The documentation is thorough, providing great credibility, and illuminating your path into even deeper study.

But don't be surprised if somewhere in these pages you begin to think of Dr. Rabe as Alan, or maybe even just Al. Don't be surprised if the author and professor becomes your friend. That's what happens when someone we respect purposefully adopts the role of humble co-learner rather than authoritative expert.

My father used to tell me there are two ways to learn—experience and example. He would go on to explain that while experience is undoubtedly the best teacher, it's also the harshest. Life is just too short to make all the mistakes ourselves. We must choose to learn from the example of others. The best of all worlds is a hybrid in which we learn through our own experience while being guided by the example of someone else.

That's exactly the opportunity *Step Outside of Your Church —Expand Your World* can provide. Dr. Rabe's research is often wrapped in Al's entertaining and compelling stories. You'll discover a rare scholar who is just as comfortable making silly faces at kids on a playground in a developing nation as he is lecturing in a U.S. graduate school. If you'll listen with your heart as you study with your mind, don't be surprised if you end up more motivated to serve more people than ever before.

Phil Tuttle, President & CEO
Walk Thru the Bible Ministries

PREFACE

Why I wrote this Book

Since becoming a Christian in October of 1970, I have been in seven different churches. Being a part of leadership in all of them, I found that the church generally is inward looking, trying to increase in numbers—numbers of attendees, baptisms, tithes and offerings, property, staff, etc., all which contribute to the church but are generally focused on that local church. For ten years I traveled the globe as a teaching missionary working in 22 different countries. More recently I have focused on three different developing countries in Asia and Africa, continuing to visit the same mission in each on a regular basis. When we focus on stepping outside of the church and into the community surrounding it, my experience has been, ***wonderful things happen***. It is important to have a stable local church. It is also important that the local church influences development in its community, region, country and worldwide. Generally, I have not observed such activity as being a high priority.

Purpose of this Book

The purpose of this book is to tell some of my story and share ideas I have learned about how transformation of society can and should be a result of church outreach in communities. Four of the five chapters have been presented live in various meetings. The material has an emphasis that leads to this end—transformation, or change of individuals, leading to broader influence that changes a community.

My Experience

From 1994 to 2003, I was the Health Officer at Food for the

Hungry International (FHI), a non-profit Christian relief and development organization, serving in over 35 countries worldwide. How ten years of world travel changed me is another story. During that same time, I was co-founder and director of the graduate International Development program within the Management Department at Hope International University (HIU) in Fullerton, California, later serving there as Dean of the School of Graduate Studies.

In 2009, my focus was as the Director and Founder of the Ministry Development Institute (MDI) at The Crossing Church in Quincy, Illinois. I continue to teach church leaders in three different countries, Cambodia, Ghana and Myanmar, as well as online courses in MDI at The Crossing. When Dr. Rufi Macagba, a Filipino surgeon, and I developed the international development program in 1994-1996, I had no sense of the direction, impact and outcome that we would see today. Thus, I am emboldened to continue teaching community development as an outreach of the church.

The Basis for these Ideas

This book is a collection of my writings to date, and of my efforts over the years to link missions and the local church to development within communities. This is not an easy task, and in many ways it borders on heresy to some, but to others it is the very process which our Lord Jesus Christ demonstrated in His ministry while on earth. I ask you, the reader, to have an open mind and to not cast aside such ideas until you at least have a general insight into the principles.

You will notice in Chapter One, *Reaching Outside of Your Church*, action steps and strategy with many examples of how God directed the lives of my wife, Linda, and I as we tried to follow Him in our earthly journey. You will gain specific insights of how you can step outside of your church. Chapter Two, *Going Beyond the Ordinary*, gives insight on how my wife and I got started in mission work which allowed us to use previously attained education, knowledge, and skills with a Biblical emphasis. In Chapter Three, *Building Partnerships*, the reader will learn how development projects should allow local participants to integrate a spiritual base along with other principles to build capacity for their community. Chapter Four, *Growing Step by Step*, indicates how missional outreach must be holistic, showing how mission agencies and personnel go through a process towards maturity. Chapter Five, *Giving Generously*, originated out of a request for me to give a paper on the subject at the National Mission Convention. It gives background for humanitarian aid but also builds the case for a biblical standard in providing aid. The *Epilogue* shows the background of Jesus starting the church in a wicked world. He sets the model for us to do the same. Finally, the poem, *The Spectacular Beijing Fifty*, is a response and glimpse of what one community of Chinese nationals experienced in a cross-cultural encounter as graduate students. Using the *Discussion Guide* individually or in a group will direct and assist you in clarifying key ideas and decisions as you plan development in the community God has given you.

As a warning, do not stop reading until you have at least read a few chapters and examined the respective Discussion Questions. The nuts and bolts of the first few chapters will give you considerable direction and detail on holistic development in local and international communities. Sometimes you may get caught in the details and not see vision for future victories. Chapter one gives strategy and plans that are adaptable at the local community level and international development program levels. The following chapters build depth and perspective. Victories happen throughout and in every step. Do not miss opportunities all along the way by stopping your dream too soon!

All of the following material supports a theme of twenty distinctives I have found to be foundational to success in community building, missions, cross-cultural work and development. Through being a missionary to being an elder in four different churches, to being a university professor and administrator, I have developed a perspective that hopefully will encourage response and action towards mission development and the church working together to follow the plan Jesus gave in Matthew 28:18-20.

Alan N. Rabe

ACKNOWLEDGMENTS

A book like this is an accumulation of the influence of so many people over five decades in various settings. Numerous names have been left out but that should not reflect the impact they have made on me and in building the Kingdom of God. Contact with such great people leads me to give thanks for the connections God has allowed in many diverse settings.

Linda, my wife, for allowing me to take countless hours each evening sitting at the computer, reviewing, and developing the ideas presented. Your partnership in life has made all the difference!

Caroline Kewney at Laser Images, Quincy, Illinois, for her tenacity in proofreading, editing and general guidance in book layout and design. Those countless hours spent are so appreciated.

Scott Schaller at scottschallerdesigns.com for cover design and the exciting years at Wednesday noon discussions on spiritual encouragement and insights.

Darrow Miller at Disciple Nations Alliance took time with me after he had spoken at Liberty University. This event led Linda and me to spend ten years at Food for the Hungry. Darrow was my direct supervisor for a number of those years.

Rufino Macagba, Jr. at Lorma Medical Center & Colleges in San Fernando City, Philippines. Our years together at Hope International University and Food for the Hungry drafting the first online course and developing the graduate International Development program set my vision and philosophy for community development.

Thanks to all those men and women I worked with over the years who are not mentioned by name. You have made an indelible imprint on my life as I sought where God wanted to use me. You are my heroes who loved me enough to direct and guide me towards service for our Master.

---------- 1 ----------

REACHING OUTSIDE OF
YOUR CHURCH

*Show me Your ways, O Lord; Teach me your paths. Lead me in
Your truth and teach me, For You are the God of my salvation; On
You I wait all the day.*
Psalm 25:4-5 (NKJV)

*Then I heard the voice of the Lord, saying, "Whom shall I send,
and who will go for Us?" Then I said, "Here am I. Send me!"*
Isaiah 6:8

My Story

My life experience has been that once an individual tastes the adventure of working in a community outside of the church, that individual gains a new vision. In October of 1970 my wife Linda and I were living in Salt Lake City, Utah. We were attending a small Baptist church on 9th South and 9th East. Linda, who had asked Jesus into her life one year before, provided an excellent example of how faith in Jesus would change my life. We also observed the faith of a few older couples who attended the Baptist church. The pastor of that church, a missionary who had recently returned from South Korea, was a compelling witness as he spoke of the importance of asking Jesus to be your Lord and Savior. Because of input from the pastor and others, that October I knelt in my bedroom and asked Jesus into my life through prayer. Transformation took place immediately and continued over the next few weeks and months.

I found myself sharing that new life with those at work and school, going to multiple weekly Bible studies, reading God's word consistently, and even planning outreach. In asking my pastor what I should do, he suggested I plan visitation in people's homes around the church. Thus, in the next six weeks my wife and I planned to visit every home in the four blocks surrounding the church. Linda and I started immediately to knock on neighborhood doors. We gave

13

each household a Chick tract (see Chick.com), then asked if they would read it. We told them we were from the nearby Baptist church and that we would drop a different tract off to them next week. The first Chick tract title, *"This Was Your Life,"* started an engaging discussion when we visited the next week. I have learned since that this tract was translated into over a hundred languages. Linda and I gained vast outreach experience in those six weeks. The neighborhood around the church was our first community.

My community expanded the next year when our family moved to Mt. Pleasant, Michigan, as I had accepted a teaching job at Central Michigan University. At another small Baptist church in the area, I began to grow and seek community outreach. This time my community included people around the church but also those I was teaching at the university. I learned that many opportunities existed with students in my classes and with those around the rural church region. After several years, I became a leader in the church. My understanding of outreach started to include physical, social, and mental, as well as spiritual activity. Playing handball with a group on a regular basis, building relationships with neighbors, students, and church attenders, as well as discussing various ideas with a group of men, all contributed.

Those years led to another outreach experience in 1977 when I was considering my first sabbatical leave at the university. Expanding community outreach was not a planned activity but it seemed to happen as I grew in knowledge of Scripture and maturity in the Lord Jesus Christ. Since international health was a contemporary topic in my profession, health sciences, I investigated what that might look like as a sabbatical leave topic. I submitted a proposal to the University sabbatical leave committee and with some changes they approved my proposal. My church pastor and leaders were a great source of encouragement to me. Our family would be heading to Haiti for a year!

The year of experience in Haiti began as a dream come true. However, it quickly turned into all work and no play. Teaching health education and practicing health care in two clinics was exciting but eventually we learned that our capacity to make this experience sustainable was not unfolding. In the clinics, at best, we were only meeting physical needs. Meeting any spiritual, mental, or social need was rather blurred and secondary. Teaching new pastors in Bible School was also about physical health. After graduation, for them to fulfill pastoral duties, they must know how to meet physical needs as people would associate them with meeting physical and spiritual needs as the witch doctors did prior to the Christian transformation. We learned the community should grow in a holistic manner, credit for our works should be given to God, and the example of service to the people must be demonstrated. We also learned community participants (insiders) need to serve with us in partnership as we (outsiders) would leave the community in the future. Lastly, our resources diminished fast as everything we were doing came from our resources. The community enjoyed things we gave them but they did not learn how to give from their heart and use local resources to make development sustainable.

A Big Step Outside My Church Ministry
    My understanding of development to transform people and communities was rapidly changing. In some obvious ways, God started to move my life away from what I wanted into what He wanted. My meaning of ministry, missional outreach, and community development started to change. In the early years of being a Christian, ministry was going to church, teaching Sunday School, being a deacon or elder, sharing the plan of salvation with an unbeliever, or simply being involved with something associated with the church.

    However, as time passed and my understanding of the Bible, church, and God matured, I found my idea of ministry changing. Ministry became more of a process of determining what God says and then doing it. It was more God-centered than church-centered. The focus was on seeking God's way, applying that to my circumstances, and doing what He wanted, sometimes in the church, but also, outside the church. The church is still God's instrument for working in this world, so it can become the encourager to get out into the world rather than remaining an organization focused on survival through metrics like numbers of attendees, baptisms, tithes and offerings, property, staff, etc.!!

    Recently, after fifty years as a Christian, the meaning of ministry has taken yet a new focus. Now ministry has less to do with what I am doing and so much more to do with a dependence on being connected to God. What I am finally realizing is true ministry only takes place when God works through me and performs His desires through this earthly vessel. That being the case, it stimulates me to know this God so very well, connect as a friend (John 15:12-15), and build a relationship through time and dialogue that allows me to function as an ambassador, (2 Corinthians 5:20) in addition to being a servant. A bond of union is acquired that can only be derived through kinship as opposed to the bond of a hired laborer. Once I have the confidence of being in the family and fully realize the Father knows my name, I have a new freedom of activity that releases me from merely doing to being a creative envoy, always open to diplomatic service that comes my way.

Such liberty is a license and release that makes one feel at home. An absolute impartial spontaneous freedom appears that allows ministry to be beyond my greatest imagination. Under this new arrangement, I do not do ministry but rather concentrate on building a relationship with the One who ultimately does the ministry despite me, but still very much through me.

Going Through the Periods of Development

In Chapter Four, we will observe the Food for the Hungry Christian agency going through characteristic periods of development. An exciting part of the Christian life is that we are all on a journey. After we start a personal relationship with God, He immediately directs us to service for Him. Peter states, *"As each one has received a special gift, employ it in serving one another, as good stewards of the manifold grace of God"* (1 Peter 4:10). As we are serving, we see needs all around us. Those needs are surely seen by us as we engage in the lives of people. As we see people with needs, we are like Jesus, *"And seeing the multitudes, He felt compassion for them, because they were distressed and downcast like sheep without a shepherd"* (Matt. 9:36). Our first step after receiving salvation from God is to sense those needs, *"therefore beseech the Lord of the harvest to send out workers into His harvest"* (Matt. 9:38). The **Relief period** is emphasized. After becoming a Christian, I immediately went to homes around our church because I realized people there had needs.

Going to those homes around the church for six weeks taught me that people were utterly lost and confused about life and wondered why they were even alive. They wanted to take responsibility for their own holistic future. They wanted to be free from a religious indoctrination that was permeating their lives. Further, many had experienced that religious indoctrination and were staunchly set against it. In the **Development period**, they wanted to become responsible for their own decisions with physical and spiritual growth in their lives. I found the same desire that year my family lived in Haiti. Haitians desired to be free from a religious dogma that permeated their country from its very founding. At that time, Haiti made a pact to the devil in order to gain their freedom from slavery under the French. As a result of the devastating earthquake on January 12th in 2010, the spiritual lacking brought by a curse was again brought up. Details of the pact can be found on the internet as we see Haitians desiring to become responsible for their own lives once the relief period was slowing. I could easily understand development was needed.

In my own life, I began to see how the **Development & Relief period** was an essential next step. People at the Salt Lake City church, as well as people in the country of Haiti, all required both relief and development. During this transition time of having their needs met, they realized they needed to take responsibility for their own future needs. This transition time is difficult because people move from a dependent culture, needing relief for the basic needs of life, towards and into a self-sustaining time when they meet their own physical and spiritual needs.

The next step of my journey was **Biblical Identity Refined**. Trying to follow this period sometimes takes many years. Building a relationship with God took many years—over those years I grew sporadically. There were tough times that I did not understand because I was striving to meet my goals and not surrendered to God's ways. Moving to Mt. Pleasant, Michigan, probably contributed the most to our family's growth. During our ten years there, we were in a wonderful well-balanced church. Strickland Baptist Church provided a great learning laboratory. There was an inward biblical maturity and an outward reach to the community around the church. The church outreach consisted of an annual summer camp, ministry at a university a few miles away, and to the world. Mission trips were happening and missionaries were commonly speaking in the church. My family and I grew under such broad spiritual development.

After spending ten years in Mt. Pleasant, Michigan, I accepted a teaching position at Illinois State University in Normal, Illinois. While attending Grace Church in Normal, Illinois, we started the next period of growth in our lives. Rubbing shoulders with great church leaders is invaluable. **Member Care & Pastoral Growth** focus was initiated at Grace in so many ways. Roger Bruehl, administrator with Campus Crusade for Christ (Cru) and currently Staff Emeritus, grew up in this church where his parents were church leaders. Serving as an elder with John Bruehl, Roger's father, and having access to Roger was an education I needed. While serving as Internship Supervisor at the church for Phil Tuttle, who was completing his master's degree at Dallas Theological Seminary, my attention was focused on how to apply ministry and community development practices within the church setting. Phil is currently President of Walk Thru the Bible in Atlanta, Georgia. Teaching second grade Sunday School with Mike and Connie Parker gave Linda and me an education in the Old Testament. Working closely with Senior Pastor John Treischmann taught me about being humble, serving the Lord in all things and gave me a vision for future learning. It was Pastor John who encouraged me to attend Liberty University even though I had no desire to leave the university where I was currently teaching. The pastoral care received at Grace was very informal—it directed me towards a formal program beyond my imagination.

The formal and informal learning I was about to participate in scared me to death. While teaching health science at Liberty University, I quickly recognized God wanted me to go beyond university walls. While teaching and working with bus kids, I got to drive the bus, visit the kids in their inner-city homes, and truly teach young children from a community outside the church. **Decentralization of Ownership** showed me how to work in a community where I had no cultural knowledge or understanding. It gave me new vision by stretching my knowledge and activity. I had to partner with minority family members, walk streets I had no reference with, and try to make sense to people who had little if anything in common with me. I learned to focus on inner-city locals who sent their children to me. They needed to learn how to take ownership for their own communities.

While teaching health science at Liberty University (LU) I was made aware of international health and ministry. This allowed me to consider new ideas and directions I had not previously considered. The **Spawning of New Specializations** allowed me to see a much bigger world than I had previously been associated with. Because of my health expertise, I was asked to travel to northern Kenya to help establish a base where students could live on a rotating basis. New directions of ministry were developing within me. In partnership with the Department of Nursing at LU, we took nursing students and health science students on short-term mission trips to Haiti. My skills and interests were growing from inner-city work to worldwide experiences. At the same time, I was working on a degree at the LU seminary. All of this promoted a big vision of God and His passion for us to serve people.

Linda and I worked with Food for the Hungry (FH) for ten years. (See website: FH.org) We traveled to twenty-two different countries presenting community development workshops (See Appendix 1). As the FH Health Officer, I strived to connect with local church-es in those developing countries with varying degrees of success. During those years I was asked to co-develop a Master's Degree in International Development at Hope International University (HIU) that could be taken online worldwide by anyone, anywhere, at any time. That degree was completed by hundreds who were in the field in over twenty-five different countries. When the former dean of the School of Graduate Studies at HIU was called to start a mission agency for children, I was asked to interview for the position. After ten years of travel to developing countries, I was getting tired. Also, I wanted to cut the cord on several development projects, but I did not want to offend. In those days, FH did not have an exact exit strat-egy because government and non-government grants compelled the partnership to sometimes last longer than best for everyone. Upon becoming dean, I could discontinue formal connections in those countries and communities. While I was dean, a graduate program with Chinese students was in progress. Also, the international development degree program grew until my retirement.

Moving from California back to Quincy, Illinois, and to The Crossing church we had formerly attended, directed me to another community. The Crossing church was a multi-site growing church and needed prepared church leaders to oversee the multi-sites being developed in various communities. Ministry Development Institute (MDI) was started consisting of a two-year online Bible program to raise up church leaders. That community of church leaders has fanned out to other churches needing leaders who cannot wait on their people to go off to school. Currently eleven multi-sites exist in three states, Illinois, Iowa, and Missouri. Campus pastors, church staff, and volunteers have taken MDI courses, and many have graduated.

MDI was then used as a basis to start a Doctor of Ministry degree program with Myitkyina Christian Seminary (MCS) in Myitkyina, Myanmar. The primary ministry of the seminary and associated mission agency was to the Lisu people, who were declared unreached at that time. The President of the seminary was Dr. Ahdee Wayezi, who was also Director of Christ for Asia Mission to the People (CAMP) mission agency there. For many years, our church had sent mission financial support to CAMP but little further contact and partnership existed. In 2013, I was asked by our church Director of Missions to make contact and build connection with this mission halfway around the world. Since then multiple groups from our church and other churches have visited annually to minister and teach in the communities, churches, Bible school, and seminary. In 2019, a group from CAMP visited us in the USA for the first time. The Lisu people group, a former unreached people in four Asian countries, have just recently become "No Longer Unreached" (PeopleGroups.org-Lisu website). Perhaps an exit strategy is evolving for us from the USA.

Community development starts small but can grow and impact worldwide. Our God is a big God and that Big God sees so much more than we do. As we follow Him and learn to humbly obey, He blesses beyond our imagination. We do not want to waste opportunities God has given us. Each opportunity He gives us is a stepping-stone to the next opportunity. Jesus said, *"If you are faithful in little things, you will be faithful in large ones. But if you are dishonest in little things, you won't be honest with greater responsibilities"* (Luke 16:10, NLT).

A Biblical Example of Development

Any biblical example of ministry outreach should come from observation of our Lord Jesus. The Bible cites many times when Jesus ministered in communities, including around the Sea of Galilee, in Jerusalem, and throughout Israel. He settled on the Sea of Galilee in Capernaum (Mark 1:21-22), attended and taught regularly in the synagogue there (Luke 4:31-37). Because the people of Nazareth rejected him, he moved to Capernaum. He chose his twelve disciples from this area too. Five of them, Peter, Andrew, James, John, and Matthew, came directly from Capernaum and all the others came from the nearby Sea of Galilee area. Although Capernaum was a small village, it was near an important road that led to Damascus. That made it a good place to meet and influence people.

I fondly remember walking into Capernaum while on a tour during 2012. It appeared to be a small sleepy town open to tourists, along the splashing waters of the sea, and where notable landmarks reminded me of many Bible stories. That experience includes Peter's house, the synagogue the centurion built and between them was a series of stone foundations showing family generations. Much could be said about Jesus using this town to focus on His public ministry. Most of the chapters in the New Testament describe the time He lived in Capernaum. This is where Jesus directed His attention to a community of men, His disciples. They were trained to reach out to communities around them.

That said, to see a direct example of development that takes place in the Bible, look at how one person and one church changed the lives of people. Perhaps the best example is where the believers were first called Christians. There is an underlying story of the apostles, Paul (also called Saul), Barnabas, and those first Christians in the Antioch church. The story shows a community and individuals who were changed for the best—community development in action (See Lesson on Barnabas).

Barnabas intercedes for a troublemaker (Acts 9:10-31). The apostles knew Barnabas as a Levite called Joseph. Acts 4:36 tells us his name literally means "Son of Encouragement." When Saul was converted in Acts 9, he was filled with the Holy Spirit (vs. 17), was baptized (vs. 18), and immediately started to proclaim Jesus as the Son of God (vs. 20). Because Saul was so powerful in proclaiming Jesus is the Christ, the Jews plotted to kill him (vs. 23). His disciples let him down from a wall during the night so he could escape to Jerusalem (vs. 25-26). The Jerusalem disciples were afraid of him (vs. 26). Barnabas took Saul to the apostles—he described Paul's salvation experience and explained how Saul had spoken out boldly in the name of Jesus (vs. 27). The disciples eventually sent Saul to Tarsus to keep him from being put to death (vs. 29-30).

Barnabas encourages a church and an individual (Acts 11:19-26). Persecution arose after Stephen's stoning and believers scattered. The believers only spoke to the Jews. Some of them started to speak about Jesus to the Greeks also (vs. 20) and a large number believed (vs. 21). Hearing about the Greeks becoming believers, the church in Jerusalem sent Barnabas to Antioch to see what was happening (vs.22). Barnabas saw the grace of God being proclaimed in Antioch as he rejoiced and encouraged them to seek the Lord. Barnabas went to Tarsus to get Saul and brought Saul to Antioch to help teach. They taught for one year with Barnabas discipling Saul. It was the first time the disciples were called Christians (vs. 26).

Barnabas turns leadership over to Saul/Paul (Acts 12:25-13:1-12). Great persecution broke out in Jerusalem, but the Word of God grew and multiplied. The Holy Spirit told the church to "set apart" Saul and Barnabas to go on the first missionary journey (vs. 2). They preached the Word of God (vs. 5) and were asked by the governor, Sergius, to share about Jesus (vs. 7). However, the magician/sorcerer, Elymas, was opposing them. He tried to keep the governor from having faith in Jesus (vs. 8). Paul (vs. 9) starred at Elymas, told him he was of the devil, and commanded him to stop opposing them. The sorcerer immediately became blind and they had to lead him around. Sergius believed in Jesus and was amazed at the Word of God. From this time on Saul is always referred to as Paul. Saul was his Hebrew name and Paul was his Roman or Gentile name—the name he used as he focused on the Gentile world.

Paul was leading because Barnabas turned leadership over to him. For the remaining time of Paul with Barnabas, we see them working together until a sharp dispute occurred (Acts 15:2, 39). Legalism of circumcision was developing in the Antioch church. Paul and Barnabas disagreed on it and were sent to the Jerusalem disciples to decide what was correct. We would later learn that they were again coworkers (1 Cor. 9:6; Col. 4:10).

Outline of a Strategy

We learn that development can start with an individual, move to a church and then on to a community. Each circumstance is different, but it usually starts with one person working with one other person—much of the time this will be an initial Bible study. As these people grow in biblical knowledge and understanding, they reach out and bring others together with them. It is amazing how simply reading through the Bible can cause change to our thinking, attitude, and behavior. Needs will be seen, and application made to a needy person or community. Change will take place based upon feedback and indicators from the focused community. Transformation of individuals occurs along the way that leads to communities being transformed. Pray, start small, and study the Bible together. Focus on needs in a group or community. Ask your church to support and pray. Build relationships and watch God direct and work! All methods of community development start with a first step which varies but, in every case, will be seeking the wisdom of Jesus and trying to follow Him. Jesus set an outline, but we fill in the details. Do not be afraid of failure—go with your gut feeling, realizing everything you try will not work. That said, step outside your church using the principles that have been outlined. The following guidelines will help.

1. Assess and select a like-minded person

The Scripture says, *"For where two or three have gathered together in My name, there I am in their midst"* (Matt. 18:20). With that special person, spend time in discussion about the Scriptures, future vision, expectations of life, why we are on earth, sharing dreams, building honesty and openness together. Two key problems in the early church were honesty and neglect. In Acts 5 we find that Ananias and Sapphira did not tell the truth and were covering this up by telling a lie. They lied to themselves, church leaders, fellow Christians and to the Holy Spirit. A second key problem is shown in Acts 6 where a certain group within the church was being neglected by leadership. The church faced these problems and a blessing resulted.

Having one or perhaps two friends to build a relationship with is essential for accountability, assistance in time of need, and to share life. Such a friend also encourages, gives honest appraisal, and helps us achieve our goals. Proverbs 18:24 says, *"A man of many friends comes to ruin, But there is a friend who sticks closer than a brother."* That kind of friend will give wonderful assistance as you grow and share life together. As your heart meshes with two or three others, God will direct in gracious unbelievable ways. Our priority is finding people who love and follow Jesus. Then build a relationship with them.

2. Pray, study, and learn together

Select a book of the Bible or a Christian book written to encourage. Try to put what you are reading into practice. It may not always work, but you have learned something if failure comes.

In my experience, a group of two to three men met for over seven years and another group of two to three men met for five years. In one group, we went through the Bible discussing a chapter each week. We finished the New Testament and went well into the Old Testament. This cell group idea is nothing new as Christ set the example.

You do not need an elaborate Bible study plan. For years, we have read the Bible, one chapter a week, and meet weekly face-to-face to discuss the reading. At the beginning we pray, but then we simply share what we have learned or have questions about in the reading. Discussion comes without any previously prepared lecture, outlines, or discussion questions.

3. Make plans to apply what you are learning

The Scripture says, *"If any of you lacks wisdom, let him ask God, who gives generously to all without reproach, and it will be given to him"* (James 1:5 ESV). It can very well be that our plans are not God's plans. In most cases, we are thinking more of ourselves than God appreciates. Wisdom is what we want so that we can see His will and do His ways. Finding His will and where He is working is dependent upon us knowing Jesus and following Him. Day 2 of *Experiencing God* tells us how to find God's will and how to see God always at work around us. The Holy Spirit and God's Word will instruct you and point you to where He is active (Blackaby, 2009:14-16). Continue to study the Scriptures as you look for what God is doing around you. The principles and distinctives outlined in future chapters should be understood as guidelines for action. In our church we sometimes call this a "D" group—D is for discipleship.

In John 15:17 Jesus gives us some direction, *"But He answered them, My Father is working until now, and I Myself am working."* Jesus was challenging the legalism of the Scribes and Pharisees because Jesus was doing only what His Father was doing. They had made the Sabbath into a bond of regulations and restrictions. When we see God working, we will expect push back from many, including "religious people." That should lead us to find activity that cannot be attributed to man. Watch for activity that is supernatural and cannot be explained or attributed to human cause. There will be sorrow, people showing great need, perhaps evil being exhibited, or certain needs for relief from some disaster. Ideas vary but your small group will discern where and in what community they might have influence. (See Lesson, "What is a Community.")

4. Start doing what you are learning

Start community outreach on a small scale so you can learn the barriers and avoid pitfalls. Reaching out to that small community is important as you want to have success early with little failure. When a few men and I started to teach a weekly Bible study at the State prison in our region, we started with the prison chaplain hand picking the men attending. We quickly gained success and within a year we were asked to do another weekly Bible study on another day with an additional group at the same prison. Within our leadership group there were a few men who dropped out for various reasons, but a few men stayed together too. Some of these Bible teachers have even gone with me to teach the Scriptures in other countries.

Avoid gaining much attention and make the beginning simple and quiet. There can be time for celebration much later but for now you just want to build good relations and good will without any fanfare or notice. We are building a reputation that can be used when God provides the bigger opportunity. Build trust, have group confidence and focus on Jesus for the goals.

5. Observe where needs exist in a new community

Build relations with a few people in that new community. Jesus spent much of his time and effort with the twelve by allowing them to observe his life in many different situations. Not everyone of us should expect to do the same thing and have the same skills. We will want to use our spiritual gifts (2 Cor. 12:4-12 ; Romans 12:4-8) without feeling we need to be everything to everyone. The interests and talents God has allowed us to develop should be used (e.g. singing, speaking, storytelling, woodworking, etc.) so those we minister to see how to use their abilities. We will work out the details with the local circumstances and needs. Usually we see community needs based upon our interests and abilities. Be careful in deciding what the new community needs. That is a job for the community.

As situations change, flexibility should be shown. Not everything tried will work, just like real life. There will be failures in the community group (insiders) and also with us (outsiders) leading the projects. Expect it and count it as a life experience to teach others how to respond. We want to teach freedom to try something new without fear of failure.

Encourage them to keep going. Much time and oversight will be needed by us (outsiders). Let's face it, Christian service is demanding. Those that have learned best from us will realize that Jesus states, *"But seek first His kingdom and His righteousness, and all these things will be added to you"* (Matt. 6:33).

6. Partner with the new community to do a community service

You are not the head of this as those in the selected community should be the ones directing the work with your guidance. You might even establish a Community Committee in this role. You are an outsider and those insiders know best. Once a group of people—a community—has been identified as potential for change, a discussion with the community leaders is needed. Outsiders can provide a service to build relationship and plan for future partnership.

The service Linda and I usually provided was a health assessment of the children in that community. We had twelve stations set up to evaluate the children—health history, vital signs, hearing, vision, dental, immunizations, spiritual relationships, etc.—and after doing the exams we would report the data to the community leaders. They would then decide what they were going to do about the problems. Of course, we would be available to partner with them to resolve the problems.

The goal for us (outsiders) is to work with those in the community (insiders) towards community betterment. There are many potential projects and needs may be obvious. We can divide a list of possible projects according to holistic components suggested later in this book, even though community development should naturally include all four holistic components.

Physical development—community clean up (picking up trash), planting flowers and trees, painting of village buildings, fixing some equipment (well pumps), building flowerpots or bird houses, building out houses, maintaining the church building, etc.

Mental development—preparing back packs for the school children, teaching health education (about nutrition, disease prevention, first aid etc.), help people complete their resumes, work with school children on homework after school, teach ESL (English as Second Language) classes, teach how to balance a checkbook, etc.

Social development—create community gardens, make home health visits, start a micro-business loan program, teach how to complete a job application and how to respond in an interview, etc.

27

Spiritual development—organize a Vacation Bible School (VBS), visit homes from which children have attended your church, give Bible lessons on contemporary topics (e.g. marriage, heaven, coronavirus), present a community concert or drama, show a Christian film in a community setting, distribute nonpartisan material for community candidates running for office, etc.

7. Reduce your involvement in the community and encourage community members to take over

Right from the start we (outsiders) must realize we are not a part of their community. We will never be as we do not live there, go to school there, eat their food, talk their talk, nor know traditions and background of past community life. Everything done should be leading towards a time when those insiders will assume the ministry in their own way. On occasions we should remind everyone that we will be leaving. This will motivate the insiders to be attentive and be extremely interested in learning.

A sense of good pride should be developing as insiders gradually become responsible for major portions of the action. The outsiders will become advisers over time. This may be true only after the outsiders officially leave the community. Outsiders will become resource people and spend less and less time in the community.

Once you have gone through this strategy cycle, determine what you have learned and reach out to a community beyond your former setting—this is usually beyond your local setting. You may teach someone or a small group within that community how to do the seven steps or you may show them by leading them through it over time. You will be amazed how they catch on. A big part of this process is watching God direct and supply what and when the next step will be.

The Future

As you gain insights, build relationships and direct people to God, you will learn so much. Expect God to give you time to develop relationships and disciple those in the community you have selected but know God most likely will also be sending you on to another assignment. You will grow as His ambassador because you have already experienced wonderful learning in a community. God wants to increase your outreach and responsibilities. He will move you on!

I will never forget leaving Haiti after a year of investing in the people there. Saying goodbye brought tears from my family and from some we built strong deep relationships with. We did some corresponding over the next few years, but it was not until six years later Linda and I started to take groups back for a few weeks each summer. We kept communication open with a few select people and planned visits. Our goal was never to be there for the rest of our lives. We were outsiders and everyone knew we would never be insiders. That same kind of knowledge and action was demonstrated in so many other settings as we moved to new opportunities through the years.

The big question is, "What do we do with what He has given us?" Do we serve the community of others or do we waste His blessings on ourselves? If we squander it upon ourselves, we will never be satisfied. Let us give it away! Jesus gives great advice when He says, *"If you cling to your life, you will lose it; but if you give up your life for me, you will find it"* (Matt. 10:39, NLT). There is no middle ground. We have two alternatives: selfishness or sacrifice. Let Christ win the battle for us and in us!

SUMMARY

Reaching out from your church looks easier when we review what has been done, but planning ahead with little assurance is challenging. The church is God's plan to restore the world. When we are open to God's direction, we make plans, but HE directs them. David says it so well, *"The steps of a man are established by the Lord; And He delights in his way"* (Psalm 37:23). Solomon also gives a wise observation, *"The mind of a man plans his way, But the Lord directs his steps"* (Prov. 16:9). The first thing to learn when considering ministry outside of the church is that God owns it. Otherwise, people, plans and projects become ours, not His. When He owns it, we can be relaxed and assured. We only need to consider the next step as we do not need to know all the steps ahead. That is faith!

Serving will be different from community to community. Our understanding and behavior after transformation will change as we grow. There is a sequence of development periods we will go through. Each period will take time, prepare us for the next period, and eventually allow us to follow our Lord in the ways He has determined. We find Biblical examples of this with Paul, Barnabas, and the disciples.

A general strategy in serving outside the church is available. Keep in mind, the church is God's organism for reaching into communities. We must view it as our *sending agent* to those in the world who desperately need help.

2

GOING BEYOND THE ORDINARY

Go into all the world and preach the gospel to all creation.
Mark 16:15

Background

It was 1977 and I had finished my first six years of university teaching, so I was determining what I would do for a sabbatical. As I pondered my interests as well as what was then a theme of current professional thinking—international health—it was a hot topic. I had never been out of the USA and doing something in another country appealed to my youthful eagerness. As I spoke with a colleague who had taken students on summer trips to the United Kingdom, I developed an even more intense desire to do something of a cross-cultural nature.

Since I was a relatively new Christian—accepted Jesus as Savior while in graduate school in October 1970—I shared a desire for doing something in another country with my pastor. He immediately encouraged me and suggested a number of places. He had recently been on a trip to Haiti with other pastors and remembered this was an annual trip. Given information, I made some contacts. After hearing replies from over a dozen different mission agencies it was apparent that I did not fit. I had no seminary training or Bible school nor did my wife and neither of us could speak a foreign language fluently. We would need to raise massive amounts of support, could only be there for a year or less and had no specific skill nationals needed. Additionally, I was not connected with the appropriate church denomination and our previous international travel was zero. I would be "high maintenance" on the field. Discouragement raised its ugly head!

All this made me think I was unsuitable for mission duty and any cross-cultural work. However, one day I received a telephone call from a mission agency who stated they had a national physician who was also a traditional healer and pastor—he was doing some

31

things in northern Haiti that might be of interest to me. Since a team of pastors was going to visit him the next summer, they wondered if I would be interested in taking such a trip. After some days of consultation and prayer, I replied "yes."

That ten-day trip to northern Haiti left an indelible impression on my mind and heart. The needs were enormous, the spiritual vitality of Haitian nationals was so appealing, and the work of the evil one was so real and obvious. A medical clinic was there where I could use my emergency medical services training and public health activity was also a possibility. My health education experience and training could be used to teach pastoral candidates skills they would need when Christian converts would come to them rather than going to the local medicine man. The national pastor/doctor seemed to like me and shared that I would do well working with him in his clinic. This was a fit!

Follow-up to a Dream

As I flew home, the excitement of this unique experience overwhelmed me. As I shared it with my wife and two pre-teen children, the gravity of the experience could not be explained. They could not grasp the picture I was painting as it was totally out of their understanding and thought process. Nevertheless, they somewhat reluctantly agreed to move to Haiti that next year in order to follow my dream. A dream that would change our lives forever was about to begin.

As we lived in Haiti that next year, we worked hard to find purpose. Working with the doctor/pastor in the clinic three days a week and teaching health education to Bible school students two days a week was taxing. Every day when we opened the clinic over 150 people were waiting for consultation. Eventually I started my own clinic in a remote area of the mountains where the same thing happened. My dream was fast starting to turn into a nightmare. We were exhausted every day. Just completing daily chores to live (e.g. cooking, washing, bathing, eating, obtaining drinking water, etc.) was difficult. The clinic work became overbearing and showed no end. It was the same hand full of problems seen over and over again— malnutrition, malaria, wounds, infections, stomach disorders, minor pain, poor teeth, parasites, skin disorders, and other preventable problems.

After leaving Haiti that year, we determined we would never return to the mission field to care for such common problems that could be preventable. Thus, our crusade to make a difference began that would lead us to a new and different type of international health. Needless to say, we had a new resolve to find a better way and one that would be sustainable.

What Then Is Included in International Health?

Paul Basch, in his well-known primer, *Textbook of International Health*, (Basch, 1999:7-8) outlines what is included in international health. In brief, but with detail, he states it is:

- principles of epidemiology and public health
- the ability to appreciate root causes of illness
- sympathetic understanding of emotional and psychological consequences which illness causes
- understanding of some economic significance of illness
- recognition of social and environmental consequences
- special consideration of similarities and differences among people in different countries
- familiarity with the structure and function of governments
- understanding the variety of healing professions
- sensitivity to the ethical aspects of research and practice
- humanitarian response to disasters and emergencies.

Basch summarizes by saying, "The popular view [of international health], shaped by the media, is understandably skewed toward immediate and dramatic themes such as epidemics and disasters rather than the unsensational struggle for rational and equitable development" (Basch, 1999:8). All these things, plus more, are generally considered as part of international health leading to development.

The World Health Organization (WHO) understood components listed by Basch and developed a definition of health that is more focused and precise. In 1947 the World Health Organization defined health as "a state of complete physical, mental, and social well being and not merely the absence of disease and infirmity" (World Health Organization constitution, 1947:29-43). With this broader definition, we can see that health is much more than the physical. For fifty-two nations to agree upon the definition for such a complex term as health, was quite a task.

From a Christian perspective, there are problems with the WHO definition (Rabe, 1993:2). One issue is that "a state of complete" being does not exist in this life. Thus, no one can be judged as healthy except that they are in a dynamic process of change. Satan is the author of confusion and deterioration, and thus has seen to it that our bodies are not in the optimal level of health, as God desires. Second, according to this concept, health is defined in only three components. As Christians we realize that a person is surely made in the image of God (Genesis 1:26). This is what makes man different from all other creation. Man has the ability to have intimate contact with the Creator through his spirit. Thirdly, health is "not merely the absence of disease and infirmity." Lacking disease symptoms or having a disability does not necessarily mean a person has good or poor health.

Health itself can be defined in various ways. Stan Rowland states "health is something much broader than the physical"— he prefers to connect physical and spiritual components to health. In his community health evangelism program (CHE) he states "the purpose of CHE is to transform individual lives physically and spiritually in local communities by meeting people at their point of need. These transformed individuals are then involved in transforming their neighbors, thereby transforming the community from the inside out" (Ram, 1995:215). There is good reason why physical and spiritual health should be examined together as they affect each other in detailed ways. The total CHE program of development depends upon the fact that health is broadly defined.

The Scriptures make note of health as a broad holistic principle. Bob Moffitt uses Luke 2:52 to define how the outreach of the church should be conducted in a "wholistic" manner. Moffitt states, "Though Jesus was divine, He was also man. His [personal] development provides a model for biblical development. Luke, a medical doctor, described Jesus' development in four domains—wisdom, physical, spiritual, and social" (Moffitt, 1995:1). The Bible states *"and Jesus grew in wisdom and stature, and in favor with God and men*" (*Holy Bible*, NIV, 1984:Luke 2:52). Moffitt illustrates by stating "Biblical development reflects **God's mind for man**, while secular development's goals are developed from **man's mind.**" Moffitt further states, "Because man's mind is rebellious by nature, it must repent—be changed to see man's condition as God sees it. If we do not know the mind of Christ, if our worldview is not found on God's word, then our goals for development will not reflect God's intentions" (Moffitt, 1995:1).

A Basis for International Development Transformation

International health provides a broad basis for international development. As we look at health in its broadest aspect, we see it is much more than doing clinic, teaching health education classes, or meeting physical needs of people in a global manner. Transformation takes place only when something has been transformed. Transformed literally means "to change the nature, function, or condition of; convert" (*The American Heritage Dictionary*, 1982). Our desire as Christian development workers is to assist the beneficiaries to change in order that they might have a better life on this earth as well as for eternity.

While the methods may be debated, Darrow Miller goes into some detail on how this transformation takes place in this world. He states in his book, *Discipling Nations*, that:

> Transformation means nothing less than radical change, in all spheres of life, as when a caterpillar turns into a butterfly. It is not merely a change in religious sentiments but a radical reorientation of a person's life. The one so transformed can then go from being soft-headed and susceptible to believing the world's lies to a tough-minded pursuer of truth. He goes from having a hard heart to a warm heart, unrighteous behavior to righteousness, and death to life. **This transformation begins on the inside, at the level of beliefs and values, and moves outward to embrace behavior and its consequences.** The gospel is so much more than evangelism (Miller, 1998:69).

Miller uses Romans 1 as the case for making such a statement. Speaking of the problems of Gentiles, Paul shows how a lifestyle develops when it is transformed without God. Unbelief is shown with its consequences. The progression develops in steps:

1. **Beliefs** are faulty   Romans 1:18-20
2. Wrong **Values** develop   Romans 1:21-23
3. Ungodly **Behaviors** result   Romans 1:24-27
4. Deathly **Consequences** come   Romans 1:28-31

Development workers must realize that "Ideas have consequences" (Miller, 1998:65). As the Bible says, "*As he [as a person] thinks within himself, so he is*" (Proverbs 23:7). As we share our ideas, transformation comes one way or the other. If shared and accepted by the beneficiaries within the truth of God, beliefs will turn to godliness, if shared based upon ourselves, the consequences will become death physically and spiritually.

Perhaps the best advice the international development worker can follow is what Basch cites as the cardinal rule for international health work. He states it "should be the same as it is for medicine: primum non nocere—first do no harm" (Basch, 1999:492). One of the things I do every time I travel to other countries is pray to God that I would do nothing to hurt others nor do anything that would embarrass my God. Thus far, God has answered such prayer to my knowledge. Certainly, any international development worker desires to help people and not hinder them. Even the most arrogant expatriate usually wants some good to come of their activity.

Another guiding principle Basch cites is " the effectiveness of international health workers, and by extension, of their programs, depends as much on understanding broad issues as on possessing narrow technical skills" (Basch, 1999:493). It is not that focused technical skills are unneeded. They are very much needed. It is to say that such technical skills need to be appraised of their adaptability to local situations, community understanding, and desire to take responsibility for oversight. I have too often seen water wells that do not work because a small washer has not been replaced to fix a pump. Various vehicles have been sitting for years because the breakdown of a small part such as an auto starter, a generator that cannot be fixed or some other common problem fixable in developed countries. While advanced technology and skills are nice, after consideration, if need be, it should be rejected, even as a gift.

Another such essential factor must be the respect for those we are working with in local settings. In order to develop such an attitude, a cross-cultural experience can be extremely helpful, perhaps even mandatory. Prejudice still exists in an inappropriately overeducated mind that breeds arrogance and superiority. A general attitude of learning must show itself in working with people, especially in cross-cultural settings. Being a learner while working in any development, local or international, will draw people to our attention as well as defuse the inevitable blunders we all make in unfamiliar settings. Being a learner establishes respect for the people we are with in ministry. Basch explains it well when he shares,

> A humble villager can do many things beyond the ability of most foreign "experts": he or she can communicate freely in their own language, and often in several; make practical and attractive objects from local materials; and survive in an often hostile environment. The untutored person may be skilled in historical tradition, agriculture, hunting or fishing, animal husbandry, music, or navigation. There is no great vacuum in their consciousness, waiting to be filled with knowledge from foreigners who may comprehend little of local problems. A reluctance to change may be based not on mulish obstinacy but on a lifetime of experience at the margin with the ever-present threat of disaster following an incorrect decision" (Basch, 1999:487-488).

It appears from Scripture that there are at least four key relationships that must be in reconciliation for a successful international development worker. According to Genesis 1, all of creation is dependent upon a proper "good" relationship with the Creator.

Day 1	light made and darkness separated	Gen. 1:3-4
Day 2	earth and seas made	Gen. 1:10
Day 3	plants and trees made	Gen. 1:12
Day 4	moon and sun made	Gen. 1:16-18

Day 5	sea animals and birds made	Gen. 1:21
Day 6	animals for the earth made	Gen. 1:25
Day 6	man made to rule over all	Gen. 1:26-28
Day 6	God saw all creation as good	Gen. 1:31

All creation was made and *it was good*. All of it was good until sin brought a change to everything, literally everything! In Genesis 3 we see broken relationships develop with all creation and God. As a result, there is no harmony in relationships between man (social), with the creation (nature), and with the Creator (God). It is rather easy to make the next step and state there is not that inner harmony necessary for one to live with our self either. Thus, each individual (self) needs to recognize their sinfulness and how that has affected their very being, especially with change in their knowledge perspective, attitude and thinking, along with activity and behavior.

Others have developed similar rationale. Elliston concludes,

> While Christians will see intermediate goals such as improved economics, roads, water systems, social structures, and justice as deserving of their very best efforts and support, they will also see the issue of reconciliation with God as having eternal significance. Three kinds of rational goals distinguish a Christian's perspective: 1) relations with God, 2) relations with others, and 3) relations with the environment. Christians seek each of these sets of relationships to be "right," recognizing that a failure in anyone affects the other two (Elliston, 1989:176-177).

Moffitt sees three of these as key components for the Christian person working in development. Moffitt states development is, "every Biblical based activity of the body of Christ, his church, that assists in bringing human beings toward the place of complete reconciliation with God and complete reconciliation with their fellows and their environment" (Vinay, 1987:236). Moffitt requires us to be actively engaged in making sure these are in harmony.

Christian Development Encompasses Transformational Distinctives

Sound development principles or distinctives are needed to form the basis of any development transformational ministry. I have observed and then used "Key Elements," or distinctives, necessary for successful Christian transformational development. These distinctives have been taught since 1996 in over twenty-five countries. During my early years working in development they have been the basis of Health Development Strategies (HDS) seminars to initiate model programs on three continents starting with three countries—Southeast Asia (Cambodia), Africa (Uganda), and Latin America (Peru). Once implemented in each of these countries, the HDS seminars were taught by nationals in surrounding communities and eventually in countries of close proximity. This is the second phase of such training where countries network by regions. We started the second phase seminars in June 2001 in Guatemala with Peruvians assisting.

Essential Distinctives
Key elements essential for appropriate and successful Christian local and international development are:

1. **Bathe the process in prayer**. (1 Thess. 5:17) *"pray without ceasing"* On many occasions we are so focused on doing, that we forget the preparation for doing. Is anything of heavenly consequence ever accomplished without the One in heaven approving and supporting?

2. **Demonstrate God's love as well as tell it**. (James 2:17) *"Even so faith, if it has not works, is dead, being by itself."* One wise man has been quoted as saying, "share the gospel with everyone and if necessary, tell them." In most cases our actions speak much louder than our words.

3. **Servant-leadership is shown**. (Matt. 20:28) *"...the son of man did not come to be served but to serve..."* When an attitude and action of service is shown, people tend to accept and follow the one serving. An example is set that is *catching*. Leadership is set by example rather than by lording it over followers.

4. **Spiritual relationship (priesthood) of believers is practiced.** (1 Peter 2:9) *"But you are a chosen race, a royal priesthood..."* Every Christian has been given gifts of the spirit to use to build up the church. When we realize this, we can allow all Chris-

tians to be instrumental in ministry. Arrogance and pride allow us to think we are the only ones who can do the best job!

5. **Holistic ministry is taught.** (Luke 2:52) *"And Jesus kept increasing in wisdom and stature and in favor with God and men."* Ministry is to the whole person. In such integrated fashion, the component parts become non-existent. Parts become almost impossible to see because of their interdependence.

6. **Community ownership is established.** (Acts 2:45) *"And they began selling their property and possessions, and were sharing them with all, as anyone might have need."* Relationships with the community are developed that make the community responsible and in charge. With this thinking, accountability is demanded by community leadership rather than by outside hirelings. Without community ownership nothing can be sustainable!

7. **Participatory methods of teaching are used.** (1 Peter 5:3 NIV) *"not lording it over those entrusted to you, ... "* With guidance, participants initiate the problems and the solutions with little bias from outsiders. Involvement is required to bring solutions. There is a major difference between the *teacher telling* as contrasted with the *student learning*. Participants must accept, internalize, and believe in the teaching so strongly that their behavior shows it by example!

8. **Community provides local resources for use in projects**. (Matt. 14:17 NIV) *"We have here only five loaves of bread and two fish ..."* Sustainability can only be reached if resources are able to be obtained by the community over time. When local resources are used, a sense of community pride exists that builds confidence.

9. **Community Committee is responsible with outside consultation**. (Proverbs 11:14 NIV) *"...many advisors make victory sure."* Broad involvement from the community brings many perspectives and increases ability for creative problem-solving. Outside consultation is only needed to further expand possible options. The community committee is best aware of community possibilities.

10. **Spiritual instruction is key component**. (Luke 8:8) *"And other seed fell into the good soil and grew up..."* Hear the word, retain it, and by persevering, produce a crop. Evangelism, Follow-up, Bible Study and Discipleship continue to be our unique part in development. When we have no spiritual plan, we may as well turn

the work over to secular groups that have more money, expertise, and resources.

Additional Distinctives
In addition to the previously mentioned essential key elements, there are additional principles that are helpful to generate successful transformational Christian development. They are:

1. **Start with small programs and let them grow naturally and slowly.** (1 Cor. 3:6) "*I planted, Apollos watered, but God was causing the growth.*" God provides success when we allow Him to chose the time for growth. Expanding should be at a pace everyone can accept.

2. **Develop collaboration and networking with partners who can fulfill missing expertise and resources.** (1 Cor. 12:14) "*For the body is not one member, but many.*" Most communities and organizations do not have the best expertise on everything. Determine what you do not have and partner with or contract with groups more knowledgeable than you are. Learn to concentrate on your strengths and not be everything to everybody.

3. **Establish a system of measurement and accountability at the beginning**. (Nehemiah 2:5) "*...send me...so that I may rebuild it.*" Starting with a well developed and agreed upon plan, monitoring progress, and continuing to rely upon established goals will keep unity of purpose and sharp focus.

4. **Select staff that are Christians and provide training to develop expertise**. (Philippians 2:2) "*...being of the same mind...*" The key ingredient in Christian development is having Christians leading by example. Non-Christians will also lead by example! The staff can be educated or trained in professional skills allowing those skills to be used in a godly manner.

5. **Staff project with people of diverse skills and interest but common goal**. (1 Cor. 12:12 NIV) "*The body is a unit, though it is made up of many parts; and though all its parts are many, they form one body...*" Philosophical unity must be focused on the ultimate goals, although different perspectives can build teamwork, unity, and broad understandings.

6. **Emphasize prevention of disease and health promotion.** (3 John 1:2) *"...be in good health..."* Our desire is to alleviate suffering before it happens rather than care for problems after they have taken form. This reduces damage and keeps disease from spreading as well as minimizing the scars of the problem.

7. **Measure results in terms of multiplication, not addition.** (John 14:12) *"...greater works than these shall he do..."* Determine success by how efforts have been reproduced in a geometric manner, rather than how one success has added to another. True development comes when each person is reproducing themselves in others and the others reproduce themselves in yet others.

8. **Demonstration projects should be developed and shared.** (Nehemiah 2:17 NIV) *"... you see the trouble we are in..."* Participants need to OBSERVE and UNDERSTAND the ultimate goal so they realize what they are working towards. Along the way, they need to discuss and comment on progress.

9. **Training takes place through home visits**. (Acts 2:46) *"... breaking bread from house to house..."* The basic unit of society is still *the family* God established in the beginning. When family members are increasingly meeting each other's needs, a wonderful synergism spreads into the community.

10. **A champion is needed to spearhead the vision.** (Nehemiah 2:5) *"...send me to Judah, to the city of my father's tombs..."* Unless one person is entrusted to keep focus, stimulate leadership, and provide a focal point of attention, everyone may depend upon everyone else to take charge. This leaves no one taking charge and the focus can easily be missed.

Concluding Remarks

Community development workers must realize that only God has the power, wisdom, and ability to understand His wonderful creation in such a manner that we can never comprehend. Only then will we discover how to build the Kingdom of God in the nations. It is about God and who He is! We need to rediscover God and the glory that only He can develop. Transformation will then come in our development efforts.

We do not need more money, more aggressiveness, more people, more time, more resources, more understanding, more networking, and more agencies. What we do need is a bigger picture of God and He will give us a bigger picture of transformation. We need a bigger picture of what transformation within community development means.

Will we take the time to seek God? Will we search His word, transform our minds, families, and hearts? Will we seek God and depend upon Him to do the transformation of families, communities, and nations? Will we treat His bride, the church, as a wonderful prize to be presented to Him? It is our decision! He is *able* and *waiting*!

SUMMARY

The desire for Christians to go beyond traditional ministry in the local church, such as programs with youth, music, education, and building maintenance, is a major step that is rather scary. Still, many believers move beyond usual church activities to a place of community development. The church goes to the people in a community as opposed to bringing people into the church for ministry. The focus for ministry outside the local church is not always widely accepted as needs in the church seem so great. Ministry with people outside the church can be at odds with traditional church thinking, and is difficult. Working with the community is usually messy. Preparing for such a venture can be misunderstood especially if working cross-culturally or in another country is being considered. We should focus on preparing to go first to a local community and then aim on going beyond. Physical, mental, social, and spiritual outreach, sometimes called holistic health, should be our target. Such development, not sums of money, meets a broad spectrum of needs that lead to transformation in the community. Certain transformational distinctives need to be followed for success.

3

BUILDING PARTNERSHIPS

You must love the Lord your God...[and] love your neighbor
as yourself
Matthew 22:37, 39 (NLT)

Background of a Problem

The church should be reaching out to communities. Holistic development is a topic that is in fashion, probably because we all believe it to be of utmost importance to the well being of any community. However, having Christian personnel who practice and promote sustainability and capacity building in local church development outreach is not common. Sustainability cannot be achieved unless capacity building with the local people within their respective communities is attained. People must take precedent over programs. On the job training can provide for capacity building that leads to sustainability, but intentional training must be in place for true success. Let us learn from examples in the real world.

One company who saw the need for capacity building is Performance Management Solutions. The objective of Performance Management Solutions is "to assist companies in capacity building by providing them with the skills, techniques and understanding of how to get the best possible performance from their staff and to make them as productive as they can be" (Performance Management Solutions website). Performance Management Solutions' core program, Performance Management Workshop, which promotes capacity building, was developed in 1992 and has been presented in twenty European countries, Africa, and the Middle East with some 2,950 participants.

Before any further examination of this problem, it is necessary to clarify what capacity building means. Performance Management Solutions states that they see capacity building as "encompassing all those activities that will assist companies in the Developing World to expand their capacity to deliver products and services in their local and regional markets" (Performance Management Solutions website). Franklyn Lisk writes in *euforic* [Europe's Forum on International Cooperation],

> Capacity building in a development context refers to a comprehensive process which includes the ability to identify constraints and to plan and manage development. The process usually involves the development of human resources and institutions, and a supportive policy environment. Ideally, it aims at improving on existing capabilities and resources and using them efficiently to achieve sustainable economic and social development (Lisk, 1996:53).

From experience in HIV/AIDS training, Family Health International states,

> The key to capacity building is working in partnership with local public and private organizations at every stage of implementation, from participatory program planning to joint evaluation and analysis, interpretation, and application of results. In addition to training nearly 200,000 people to deliver HIV/AIDS services, FHI has built capacity by providing technical assistance in a way that gives local counterparts opportunities to learn on the job (Family Health International website, 2002:1).

As we study public private partnerships (PPPs), we can observe that such entities need to exist and function for successful capacity building. Partnerships between stakeholders are crucial for capacity building if sustainability is to occur as sustainability can only be accomplished if local personnel are involved.

> For the Carl Duisberg Gesellschaft [CDG], a joint endeavour of industry and government which goes back more than 50 years, the discussion on the role of public private partnerships (PPPs) in development cooperation is a welcome enrichment of the developmental debate. Indeed, the CDG with its more than 1,000 members—mostly institutions, companies and individuals in the private sector—saw itself as a

public-private partnership long before the term was coined (Reuter, 2002:12).

CDG cites the following reasons why PPPs need to exist:

- Local companies [can be used] as project partners
- Companies [have expertise to be used] as a training venue
- Using the know-how of the private sector
- Providing training programmes for private sector companies
- Making services for companies available (Reuter, 2002:13).

As an example, we can look at my experience conducting two week-long workshops in 1998 and 2000 in Chaclacayo-Lima, Peru. Focus was on community leaders, churches, and families building partnership. Food for the Hungry provided the Vision of Community training program for Child Development Programs. Vision of Community goals emphasizing partnership between community leaders, churches and families brought about: (Appendix 1)

- Leaders increasingly solving community problems,
- Churches increasingly reaching out, and
- Families increasingly meeting each other's needs.

CDG states PPPs benefit companies in several ways:

- Preparation and securing of investments [otherwise not available]
- Promotion of export projects and acquisition of orders [to develop relationships]
- Promotion of company cooperation
- Improving competitiveness [to stimulate high standards]
- Secure market access by environmental and social standards (Reuter, 2002:14).

Demonstration of such public private partnerships (PPPs) brought further success as I completed a workshop in Manila, Philippines, in November 2001. Our plan was exceeded when we integrated lessons from Community Health Evangelism (CHE) with Food for the Hungry Vision of Community linked with local goals to introduce a previously developed Child Health Strategies booklet. The outstanding booklet was paid for by a generous donor. The booklet addressed the two hungers, physical and spiritual, and prompted the community to develop their God given potential, defined cooperatively by two organizations and the local community.

Capacity building in non-governmental organizations (NGOs) like churches has been a challenge as much talk has taken place but the action is many times missing. A real-world working group of interested practitioners have come together in the past few years to discuss just this problem. Communitybuilders.nsw (in New South Wales, a southeastern Australian state, including the capital, Sydney) is a group working together to strengthen communities and can be located on the internet at http://communitydevelopment.org.au. It is clear from this listing that capacity building for Nongovernmental Organizations (NGOs) is being talked about, but action seems to be lacking. Communitybuilders.nsw has compiled key issues that need to be discussed to provide for capacity building in communities. The main issues are summarized—they provide common strengths to assist boards and management committees of NGOs, especially Christian groups. Reasons for building greater relationships with local participants in the community include:

> They have local knowledge, they are trusted and have credibility, they have specific objective industry knowledge, they are accessible and resourced, they are able to critically evaluate NGO issues, they adopt a Board and Management Committee support role, and they have the ability to develop and broker tailored solutions to issues…Other issues identified include resourcing, training/support content and the need for flexibility in the delivery of programs (Communitybuilders website, 2001:1).

I found the capacity building insights from Communitybuilders to be so helpful. A challenge to action in capacity building was met in Kampala, Uganda, upon completion of two Child Development Program workshops I directed in 1997 and 2001. The key reasons for success were: local people approved the workshop content, participants were from local child-focused agencies, they knew the needs and resources within the communities, most were leaders within local NGOs, and all realized that flexibility is essential in implementing ideas in communities.

In summary, we find NGOs, private companies, and government agreeing that project sustainability and local personnel capacity building is essential for successful management in development. Local personnel (insiders) need to be empowered and involved in decision making from the start, as it is they who will live there and foster any benefits. In short, **insiders** must be transformed so they can complete the work started by those not living in the community (**outsiders**). Outsiders must decrease their influence and remain at a low level of control. Even though training sessions do take place, local participants do not normally have the power to establish sustainability until outsiders diminish their influence. A transformation and an understanding are essential for the insider to grasp the appropriate vision. Much of the time outsiders simply want to "get the job done" and do not see beyond immediate plans.

During the ten years I led Health Development Strategies seminars in various developing countries, I always had a lesson near the end of the week-long workshop that taught exit strategies. In other words, from the beginning of the partnership everyone understood that there was a time coming when the insiders would take over and the outsiders (my agency and me) would reduce efforts and eventually not be involved. It was planned!

The lesson on exit strategy included:
- how we had started with a partnership,
- expectations or goals of insiders and outsiders,
- anticipation that over time insider's efforts would increase and outsider's efforts would decrease,
- a timeline of changing responsibilities during three to five years in the partnership process,
- focus and description on how to utilize local resources whenever possible, and
- a listing of responsibilities of insiders and outsiders.

I would usually ask the Director of the Program (an outsider) to present the lesson so all participants could hear and be assured of responsibility being shifted. This would remind the participants (insiders) that they would eventually become owners of the project. Thus, they needed to be diligent in understanding and preparing for that day to come. In almost every instance, reluctance was shown by the insiders but a new attention to accountability was gained.

The goal of this book is to provide intentional principles and practices that lead to sustainability in capacity building for personnel in local community development.

Transformational Development in Capacity Building

Transformation means change. Miller says, "Transformation means nothing less than radical change, in all spheres of life…" (Miller, 1998:73). The key ingredient in capacity building for Christian community development is for transformation to take place within the participants. Myers states, "There is a tendency for development practitioners to tune out the spiritual" (Myers, 1999:193). For participants to develop the knowledge, attitudes, and action obtained from a Biblical worldview, it is necessary that the local management team understand and be able to apply scriptural principles. It is absolutely essential for those who are to successfully oversee and continue a work to be those who have a relationship with the One True Creator God who made everything. It is only God who is able to provide that which is ultimately needed—a new look at the world from a heart that is genuine, sincere, and in right relationship with the Creator.

Ajulu concludes this thought by saying, "The way to empowerment advocated in the Bible involves dealing with human sin as central to human greed and self-centeredness, the underlying cause of many problems under discussion here" (Ajulu, 2001:13). A change or transformation allows participants to "…*throw off everything that hinders and the sin that so easily entangles…*" (Hebrews 12:1, NIV).

Myers outlines two reasons why he prefers to use the term "transformational development" as an alternative to the more traditional "development" term. He cites the traditional term development is:

> …heavily loaded with past meaning, not all of which is positive. When most people think of development, they think of material change or social change in the material world. Second, development is a term that many understand as a synonym for Westernization or modernization. Too often this understanding of development is associated with having more things (Myers, 1999:3).

Such traditional understanding of development is not what many of us think to be the best. There is more to development than beneficiaries simply receiving material things to make their lives easier or development managers holding the authority to give resources at their will.

Myers goes on to say transformational development shows concern for human life in material, social, and spiritual ways so that choices that are made reflect the core values and beliefs of God. Some might call this "Christian witness" in which demonstration of beliefs will guide our activity. A Christian identity and understanding should shape our development activity. Myers states,

> My Christian identity and my understanding of my faith shape my view of what development is for and how it should be done. Part of that understanding is my conviction that the best news I have is the knowledge that God has, through his Son, made it possible for every human being to be in a covenant relationship with God. We need only say yes to this offer. To not share this news, to not yearn that everyone might share what was given to me through no merit of my own, would be wrong in the deepest and most profound sense. Christian witness is the term that I use to describe this news that Christians are compelled by love to share (Myers, 1999:3-4).

The Christian witness Myers speaks of is the outer declaration of the inner gospel displayed by life, word, and deed. Development workers should show Christian character and understanding by their walk, talk, and actions. Active demonstration of these traits will be most instrumental in teaching capacity building principles important for sustained development once the outsider is gone. "That is why engaged, respectful relationships are so important to transformational development" (Myers, 1999:138). We cannot underestimate the need for development beneficiaries to obtain this understanding and life focus.

Elliston makes a strong case for development training that will make a decisive difference in how development workers will foster sustainability. In explaining why a spiritual base is necessary for

51

instruction of development workers, he states,

> The spiritual formation serves as the base on which all else rests. The spiritual formation provides the value, worldview, and being base, both for learning and ministry. The insistence on the establishment of a strong spiritual formation base provides one of the key distinctives of the Christian relief and development worker…without a dynamically growing spiritual base, the whole lifestyle, ethics, values, and direction of the enterprise will likely go awry (Elliston, 1989:244).

The greatest factor in sustainability of a Christian worldview is perhaps how and what instruction took place with the local development worker. If little or cursory integration of Biblical truth is in the initial training of a development worker, the future use of spiritual wisdom in future decision making and training will be minimal too.

Ben Holman, former President of Food for the Hungry, answers the question, "Is it right to change people's culture when you go into a community to help them?" What he says about Food for the Hungry is what most Christian development workers would think and hopefully practice.

> Food for the Hungry isn't about changing cultures or stripping people of their heritage. We're about finding a need, accepting an invitation to help, and offering something more—Eternal life through Jesus Christ.

> Instead of changing cultures, we're about changing hearts—transforming communities with the love of God.

> So what does that really mean to those we serve?

> It means nutritious food and safe water to families hurt by drought. It means long-term solutions that will help long after Food for the Hungry is out of the picture. And it means changed hearts.

> There's just no way around it, really. When you meet Christ and experience His mercy, you just can't help but be transformed (Holman, 2002:2).

For sustainable capacity building to take place in any community, spiritual integration must be part of the total development program which includes training, planning, implementation, and evaluation. Changing the hearts of the participants to reflect the character of Jesus Christ is the necessary transformation in capacity building that will lead to true sustainability. Without this intentional transformation or change of participants' beliefs, communities and individuals will never experience the best development results. Capacity building will be limited, beneficiaries will experience partial results, and management will be restricted, unless transformational development is demonstrated to declare the God to depend on and live by.

Distinctives for Successful Christian Community Development

For a decade I facilitated Health Development Strategy seminars on three continents. What has developed, through experience, observation, and counsel, are ten essential and ten additional transformational distinctives that are necessary for successful community development activities (Rabe, 2001:10). With each principle is a key Bible passage to emphasize the theme of the respective principle with an Application Example following. These practices can be the guiding principles for management of capacity building in community development. Many are common sense, but common sense does not guarantee application. To realize any benefit, management must be intentional about integrating each principle into the developmental activities at every level and stage. Of the ten essential distinctives provided, five relate directly to capacity building. Those five are titled Key Distinctives for Capacity Building and will be explained later in this section with background and application.

Essential Distinctives

Key elements essential for appropriate and successful Christian local and international development are:

1. **Bathe the process in prayer**. (1 Thess. 5:17) *"pray without ceasing."* Application Example: Before going into the community each day to do a neighborhood cleanup, our group met to pray for those we would meet and build relationships with.

2. **Demonstrate God's love as well as tell it**. (James 2:17)

"*Even so faith, if it has not works, is dead, being by itself.*" Application Example: While picking up trash in the community, various residents would ask what we were doing. We would say, "Because of the love that Jesus showed for us, we want to show that love to others."

3. **Servant-leadership is shown**. (Matt. 20:28) "*…the son of man did not come to be served but to serve…*" Application Example: Helping a widow repair her screen door caused her to come to church the next weekend.

4. **Spiritual relationship (priesthood) of believers is practiced.** (1 Peter 2:9 NIV) "*But you are a chosen race, a royal priesthood…*" Application Example: When volunteers were asked why they were painting a neighborhood house, they would explain what Jesus meant to them in a few thoughtfully worded sentences. Each of the volunteers knew Christ personally and intimately.

5. **Holistic ministry is taught.** (Luke 2:52) "*And Jesus kept increasing in wisdom and stature and in favor with God and men.*" Application Example: While visiting in homes, we were constantly looking for ways of helping both physically and spiritually.

6. **Community ownership is established.** (Acts 2:45) "*and they began selling their property and possessions, and were sharing them with all as anyone might have need.*" Application Example: When doing work in any community, we always had people from that community working with us.

7. **Participatory methods of teaching are used.** (1 Peter 5:3 NIV) "*not lording it over those entrusted to you,…*" Application Example: When teaching others how to fix a well pump, community members would do much of the work as we assisted.

8. **Community provides local resources for use in projects**. (Matt. 14:17 NIV) "*We have here only five loaves of bread and two fish …*" Application Example: Any items needed to plant, maintain or harvest the community garden were purchased in that community or in a nearby location.

9. **Community committee is responsible with outside consultation**. (Proverbs 11:14 NIV) "*…many advisors make victory sure.*" Application Example: When asked to decide on the location of a community outhouse, the question was directed to the commu-

nity committee even though the missionary outsider already had an opinion.

10. **Spiritual instruction is key component**. (Luke 8:8) *"And other seed fell into the good ground…"* Application Example: Before, at noon, or afterwards, a brief meeting was scheduled for a devotion leading to thanksgiving to God.

Additional Distinctives

In addition to the previously mentioned key elements, there are additional principles that are helpful to generate successful transformational Christian development. They are:

1. **Start with small programs and let them grow naturally and slowly.** (1 Cor. 3:6) *"I planted, Apollos watered, but God was causing the growth."* Application Example: When teaching handwashing to children who had no running water, over time, community leaders started to plan how to pipe water to the school so children would be healthier.

2. **Develop collaboration and networking with partners who can fulfill missing expertise and resources.** (1 Cor. 12:12-14) *"For the body is not one member, but many."* Application Example: While holding a clinic in a community, as individuals needed advanced consultations, local community nurses in the group would send those needing deeper evaluation to the hospital.

3. **Establish a system of measurement and accountability at the beginning**. (Nehemiah 2:5) *"…send me…so that I may rebuild it."* Application Example: While doing physical exams on school children, standards were developed for when to refer children elsewhere for advanced eye, hearing, teeth and infection problems.

4. **Select staff that are Christians and provide training to develop expertise**. (Philippians 2:2) *"…being of the same mind…"* Application Example: While starting a micro-business loan program, an accountant was needed. The first criteria for selecting that person was their relationship with God. Next, their professional skills would be considered. One time a person in the church was selected and sent off to learn basic accounting procedures before working in the micro-business loan program.

5. **Staff project with people of diverse skills and interest but common goal**. (1 Cor. 12:12 NIV) *"The body is a unit, though it is made up of many parts; and though all its parts are many, they form one body..."* Application Example: Members of the Community Committee were selected because of their different abilities, but each of them always had the health of the community in mind. People with different skills—carpentry, bookkeeping, healthcare, legal, banking, parenting, teaching, etc. were chosen—this helped provide perspective.

6. **Emphasize prevention of disease and health promotion**. (3 John 1:2) *"...be in good health..."* Application Example: After doing a child health assessment in a village, a presentation was made to the community leaders on better water management.

7. **Measure results in terms of multiplication, not addition**. (John 14:12) *"...greater works than these shall he do..."* Application Example: While teaching prevention of measles to children and teachers, it was decided that upon completing the course, each participant should instruct two others in their respective neighborhoods.

8. **Demonstration projects should be developed and shared**. (Nehemiah 2:17 NIV) *"... you see the trouble we are in...."* Application Example: A class was taught in how to make a roof-top garden. After successfully learning the process, students would have others visit and watch a demonstration of what they had learned.

9. **Training takes place through home visits**. (Acts 2:46) *"...breaking bread from house to house..."* Application Example: After teaching a lesson at church on the Lord's Supper, church leaders would visit homes and take part while the house leader presented communion.

10. **A champion is needed to spearhead the vision.** (Nehemiah 2:5) *"... send me to Judah, to the city of my father's tombs..."* Application Example: When planning a community irrigation project, a farmer in the community was taught about irrigation in a nearby community. He could then return to his community and direct the needed project. A *champion* should be enthusiastic, informed, and accepted by those he or she will lead.

Key Distinctives for Capacity Building

Of the ten essential distinctives that provide for successful Christian community development, five have very intentional focus on capacity building in management of local development personnel. Holistic ministry, community ownership, participatory teaching, local resources, and the community committee are critical key components for capacity building that leads to sustainability. Each will be discussed with background and application.

Holistic ministry is taught. (Luke 2:52) "*And Jesus kept increasing in wisdom and stature and in favor with God and men.*" Ministry is to the whole person (mental, physical, spiritual, social) in such integrated fashion that component parts become non-existent. Parts become almost impossible to see because of the interdependence.

Transformational development requires participants to evaluate their spiritual condition because the spiritual component is inherently part of the whole person. "A holistic biblical position holds that no one is intrinsically good or capable of consistently doing good, because of the principle of human sin (Mark 10:18; Luke 18:19; Romans 3:9-12; 23)"(Ajulu, 2001:13). This fact is more clearly understood by those in the developing world because many in the developed world have demoted spiritual things to the weak, mystic, and fanatics. In years of teaching, I have never had a student in the developing world deny the importance of the interdependence of physical and spiritual components.

Physical and spiritual ministry is important. Sometimes the term "holistic" can cause us misunderstanding. The word "holistic" comes from the Greek Holos meaning whole, wholly, or complete. It is a biblical word used to express completeness or totality as in Matthew 5:29-30; John 7:23; 9:34. Many people debate whether it should be spelled "hole" or "whole" but either way is possible. Holism with the "h" is the Greek-based spelling and wholism with the "w" is the anglicized version. Sometimes it is confused with the word holy, but this is not the same meaning. Whatever the case, the issue is that ministry should be total and complete. That is, it should not be secular or sacred, work or ministry, spiritual or physical. That result is a split Christian mind followed by a separated behavior.

Such dualistic notion dominates much Christian thinking today. Paul had to work with the Colossians who had excellent teaching from Epaphras (Col. 1:7) but still needed to be reminded that Christ was Supreme over everything (Col. 1:18), including heaven and earth, visible and invisible, thrones or powers, rulers or authorities (Col. 1:16-17). Landa Cope, a YWAM trainer, presents it well by saying,

> The Gospel of the Kingdom that Jesus taught and that the early church multiplied and built on the foundation of was the entire teaching of God to Israel through Moses and the prophets. It was a message that dealt with sin, and salvation, with heaven and hell, with prayer and spiritual warfare. But it was also a message that dealt with God's desires for justice in government, equity in economics, the righteous use of science and technology, communication, family, the arts, and all of life" (Cope, 2001:2).

The split view of the world relieves the split-minded Christian from concern for social issues as they concentrate only on spiritual issues. On the other hand, teaching holistic ministry means to teach that every **thought** (2 Cor. 10:5) and every **thing** (Col. 1:18) is understood to be under the authority of Christ. In other words, all four holistic components, mental, physical, spiritual, social, are essential.

Community ownership is established. (Acts 2:44-45) *"Believers sold property and possessions and were sharing them with all as anyone might have need."* Relationships with the community are developed to such degree the community knows they are responsible and in charge. With this thinking, accountability is demanded by community leadership (insiders) rather than outsiders. Without community ownership nothing can be sustainable!

Local people must be empowered for sustainability to occur. Ajulu makes a detailed case for the empowerment of people when she states, "Empowerment of people must lead to creation of a caring community characterized by neighborly love, stewardship and justice, all central to a biblical approach" (Ajulu, 2001:13). It is only when we enable individuals and communities that they can become self-reliant and able to capture their God-given dignity and abilities. Conclusion is that "just and caring communities and eventually nations can only result as people learn how to use their given resources for poverty alleviation and sustainable development…" (Ajulu, 2001:13). For example, the Pocomchi people of central Guatemala grasped development ideas only after they learned they were responsible for teaching and applying the principles I was sharing.

Participatory methods of teaching are used. (1 Peter 5:3 NIV) "…*not lording it over those entrusted to you,…*" With guidance, participants initiate the problems and the solutions with little bias from outsiders. Involvement is required to bring solutions. There is a major difference between the teacher telling as contrasted with the student learning. Participants must accept, internalize, and believe in the teaching so strongly that their behavior shows it by example!

Applying the participatory approach to teaching may be difficult for some as it requires lessons to be LePSAS oriented with focus on the learner, not on the teacher. (LePSAS is an acronym used to mean Learner-centered, Problem-posing, Self-discovery, Action-oriented, and Spirit-guided.) I have taken many ideas for various participatory development lessons from experiences and synthesized them with resources from selected agencies. Agencies include Save the Children, Teaching Aids at Low Cost (TALC), World Neighbors, and Child-to-Child Trust with lessons and ideas, especially on child-to-child approach. After presenting participatory lessons to numerous groups on three continents, I am convinced that the best learning takes place when students are involved. Myers suggests the participatory approach as being the best means to facilitate local poor to discover what they know is valuable (Myers, 1999:173-174).

The International Institute for Environment and Development (IIED) in 1988 started publishing a periodical three times per year titled Participatory Learning and Action Notes (PLA Notes) that reaches over 10,000 readers in 47 countries. The material is copyright-free, from the field, and is also on CD-ROM (International Institute website). Material that can be found consists of over 2,500 participation related documents.

An additional and extremely popular contemporary program titled Community Health Evangelism (CHE) also requires and shows participatory involvement in each lesson. Groups are asked to do something, then discuss what happened and determine how that activity could be implemented in respective communities. Almost all Christian missionary agencies currently use part or all of CHE when working in communities. Most lessons can be obtained online at: http://www.neighborhoodtransformation.net for urban CHE or for developing countries at: http://www.chenetwork.org. Neighborhood Transformation, LifeWind International, Medical Ambassadors, Micah Network and other groups sponsor and use these participatory activities for excellent success. I have participated in urban workshops in the USA and taught CHE training in developing countries and find it to be extremely valuable for transformational development.

Community provides local resources for use in projects. (Matt. 14:17 NIV) *"...We have here only five loaves of bread and two fish."* Sustainability can only be attained if resources are able to be obtained by the community over time. When local resources are used, a sense of community pride exists that builds confidence.

Use of local resources also tells the community that "they can do it" and builds a sense of independence and self-reliance. In January of 2001, my wife and I were teaching a Health Development Strategy seminar in Uganda. One part of it was to teach how to do child health assessments. Since we had not brought along enough tongue blades for the oral examination, questions came about how and where they could purchase them. Cost was prohibitive so a discussion transpired about alternatives. One person stated, "Each child should bring a spoon from home that will be used by the health worker when an oral exam is done." The group was proud and was excited to do the work. To this day, they use spoons for the oral exam! Answers to needs must come from within the community.

Community committee is responsible with outside consultation. (Proverbs 11:14 NIV) *"...many advisors make victory sure."*

Broad involvement from the community brings many perspectives and increases ability for creative problem-solving. Outside consultation is only needed to further expand possible options where expertise is lacking inside the community. The community committee is best aware of community possibilities.

In the numerous Health Development Strategy (HDS) seminars we have taught over years around the globe, we always try to have a "Reflection & Consultation" time at the end so participants might discuss anything that is on their minds. Of all the questions that are asked, there is one category that is most common: staff responsibility in the community. Questions include, "What if the community leaders do not want to do what I tell them?" or "How do you handle disagreement between leaders?" or "What if the community does not have essential resources for a project?"

The answer is always the same. You let the community committee decide. The community committee is made up of six to nine representatives from the local community and should take responsibility for all parts of the projects. Outsiders are for consultation only! Even if insiders do not have the resources, they can decide alternative ways to do the project, look for resources, visit a nearby community to see how they handle a similar problem, or be assisted by you, the outsider, to find the resources (not for you to give the resources to them). Every piece of this activity will be building capacity that will lead to sustainable development.

Conclusion

A major problem is facing management of sustainable holistic development. That problem is that such programs and projects cannot be sustainable unless capacity building of local personnel is at the heart of training. The same problem exists in all development but in holistic development capacity building is even more crucial because of the interdependence of all activities. Building a relationship with the people being trained is as important as forming technical skill. Those being trained who will also teach others must embrace distinctives that lead to transformation. For any holistic development project to succeed, the goal must include capacity building that leads to transformation of local participants being trained who will continue the work. All distinctives will assist for success.

SUMMARY

Good management of sustainable holistic development requires capacity building of local participants who will be responsible for continuing the efforts once outsiders (those not living in the community where they are working) have left the community. A partnership between public and private organizations that link with local community leaders is needed. In many cases, development projects started by outsiders lack such capacity building and are simply focused on completing project goals. It is not common to have local participant capacity building as a goal for most projects. This book suggests intentional principles necessary to provide capacity building that leads to sustainability. Transformational development of local workers is a top priority in capacity building. Transformation provides opportunity for local participants to obtain a Biblical worldview and integration that will be used as a spiritual base for the future. The twenty principles needed to build capacity are mentioned in this section including holistic ministry, community ownership, participatory teaching methods, use of local resources, and a community committee. These principles can guide any development project and a worker who is focused on sustainable transformational development.

———— **4** ————

GROWING STEP BY STEP

He who began a good work in you will bring it to completion
Philippians 1:6 (ESV)

Introduction

Development is a word that brings to mind preconceived meanings that probably cause some to be uneasy and others to consider a very narrow view of social change. Most missionaries and mission agencies either consider themselves working in development or not, based upon their interpretation of physical, spiritual and social focus. Many people will think of a social gospel, cultural change, or giving of things as a substitute for preaching of the gospel. Others may think development is transplanting western Christianity into non-western cultures. Some may feel development is bringing people groups into modern times so people will use electricity, gasoline autos and tractors, radio, etc.

Perhaps, another perspective of development is whether the agency has a holistic vision and meets the spiritual and physical needs of the indigenous groups being targeted. Transformational development is a term Myers discusses. Myers states, "I use the term transformational development to reflect my concern for seeing positive change in the whole of human life materially, socially, and spiritually" (Myers, 1999:3). This is the type of development discussed in this book.

The purpose of this chapter is to review selected development trends in contemporary community outreach, draw attention to key activities, and suggest future action. A case study will be used as an example to show how one agency and its personnel changed over time to allow development to be fully implemented.

What is Development?

Several development perspectives exist and should be considered in an effort to synthesize ideas that will best apply to individual circumstances. David Korten, Director of People-Centered Development Forum, contrasts people-centered development with economic growth-centered development, which many Western governments promote. He defines development as "a process by which the members of a society increase their personal and institutional capacities to mobilize and manage resources to produce sustainable and justly distributed improvements in their quality of life consistent with their own aspirations" (Korten, 1990:67). He sees development as a process, capacities, sustainable, and just and consistent with aspirations of the targeted group. It is a continuing process of empowering communities to continue on their own within an expectation of the community rather than within preconceived outside notions. He even states that there is a spiritual component that is necessary for transformation, but the spirit may be decided upon by the community rather than an absolute as in Christianity. Although full of good ideas, this kind of development may not be what most community projects have in mind.

Robert Chambers, author of the book *Whose Reality Counts? Putting the First Last*, shows how poverty entraps the poor and states current development is represented in five words: well-being, livelihood, capability, equity, and sustainability (Chambers, 1997:10). He sees development as an interdependent process made up of key components providing synergism with each other. The problem is that Chambers does not address the spiritual dimension, the good in people, the bad in people, and the perception people may have that they are fine in poverty.

Jayakumar Christian, an experienced Indian development worker in World Vision, sees the poor trapped inside four systems of disempowerment: cultural system, social system, spiritual/religious system, and personal system (Christian, 1994:4). The social system reinforces the powerlessness of the poor by exclusion and exploitation and by the heavy hand of the rich and those desiring to do good. Those who are not poor tend to encourage the poor to be poor. Through it all, a basic practice of rebellion against God forms as a main ingredient. Christian emphasized a key identity of the poor, which illustrates why it took forty years to get the experience of Egyptian slavery out of the minds of Israel before a nation could be built in the promised land. A culture of poverty is real.

Perhaps true development is best understood when we look at what Christian and Miller, along with Myers, all see as a battle against a "web of lies" in which the poor are caught (Christian, 1994:264; Miller, 2001:68-73; Myers, 1999:77-80). A few examples of lies might be:

There is no tomorrow.

Truth, if it exists at all, is unknowable.

Human life has no value.

Miller states such a web must be broken in three ways: preaching the gospel, renewing minds, and discipling nations. Based upon Romans 1:16; Ephesians 2:1-6; Mark 12:29-30; Romans 12:2; 2 Corinthians 10:5; 1 Peter 1:1-13; John 8:32; Matthew 28:19-20; a case can be made (Miller, 2001:70-72). The Hindu belief system is most enlightening of this kind of thinking, but it permeates all religious beliefs even to the infiltration of Christian thought. Christians discuss topics like selfish desires versus group benefit, levels of Christian maturity, the earning of wealth, personal responsibility for your station in life, past good or bad that determines the present level of spirituality, etc.

Maybe a best case is made by Ravi Jayakaran, an Indian practitioner of PLA (Participatory Learning and Action) methods, when he cites poverty as a lack of freedom to grow in four areas cited by the apostle Luke in Luke 2:52. One cannot grow in mental (wisdom), physical (stature), spiritual (favor with God), and social (favor with man) dimensions because of this entrapment (Jayakaran, 1996:14). The cause of poverty and thus the need for development is in people, not in concepts, the system, culture, or corruption. Further, everyone is a sinner and is sinned against so that no matter where you are in the levels of wealth, you are held in bondage. God is the one true creator and the final judge.

A contemporary and very promising view of Christian community development has been implemented and practiced by the CHE model founded by Stan Rowland. "The acronym CHE may stand for community health evangelism, community health evangelist, community health education, or community health educator" (Rowland, 1995:233). I have participated in and taught CHE for many years while Health Officer in Food for the Hungry International and found it to be very relevant. Rowland explains what CHE is by stating:

> Community health evangelism (CHE) is a strategy to restore harmony or wholeness in individuals. The purpose of CHE is to transform individual lives physically and spiritually in local communities by meeting people at their point of need. These transformed individuals are then involved in transforming their neighbors, thereby transforming the community from the inside out. This is multiplied to other areas, eventually transforming an entire country for Jesus Christ (Rowland, 1995:215).

CHE teaches "transformational development—development that transforms people, groups, communities, governments, and countries from the inside out" (Rowland, 2001:73). CHE supports a heavy emphasis on local community committee direction. CHE programs "feel that the individual members of the committees are important, and we need to spend time training and discipling each of them. 'Vision is caught, not taught,' as an old saying goes" (Rowland, 2001:75). The CHE approach is holistic, has a Bible base, promotes living in harmony with self, God, others, then nature, emphasizes church and community, and encourages grass-roots development (Rowland, 1995:chapter 14).

Why then development?

We have looked at a number of thoughts on how development might be viewed to combat poverty and embrace needs in the world and build the kingdom of God. Poverty is complicated and so are the means to counter it—such as development. Development must embrace all elements of life. However, at some point we will see development of poverty-stricken peoples to be a perception of the observer. How we view poverty, notice needs of people, wrapped with our former experiences and teaching of development can, but need not, set how we embrace working with people in all areas of life. We must have our eyes open and be aware of holistic needs by people, especially the poor.

Background—A Development Agency Case Study

Food for the Hungry International (FHI) is a non-profit, Christian, relief and development organization dedicated to compassion ministry of meeting holistic physical and spiritual needs of the hungry with the world's poorest of the poor. Founded in 1971 by Dr. Larry Ward, FHI operated on the principle that the hungry die one at a time; therefore, they can be saved one at a time. Dr. Ward had previously been a managing editor at *Christianity Today* and Vice President of Information Services at World Vision. The name "Food for the Hungry," was given by Dr. Ward in reflection upon Psalm 146:7-8 (NIV), "*He upholds the cause of the oppressed and gives food to the hungry. The Lord sets prisoners free, the Lord gives sight to the blind, the Lord lifts up those who are bowed down, the Lord loves the righteous.*"

FHI's early history and formation can be divided into five major eras:

1971-1980	Founding and relief period
1981-1985	Transition period with increased emphasis on development
1986-1993	Development era with significant relief efforts
1993-2000	Creation of the Corporate Identity with Vision of Community (VoC) as the impact statement giving focus to FHI's worldwide work
2001-2010	Staff development period with emphasis on the VoC tree and human resources (Wheeler 2003:16-19).

During the founding period, FHI was directly focused on relief and based in the United States. Within this time, some long-term development efforts were tried, but the importance of promoting long-term development was just being realized. With this discovery, there became a division where the U.S. based office became known as FH, Inc. and the international office and field offices became known as FHI.

A Transition Period was brought about in 1981 when headquarters was chartered in Geneva, Switzerland, as an international relief and development organization. For the next four years most FHI programs started by entering a country to conduct relief work and then making the transition to development. A second National Organization (NO) was established in Japan (JIFH) in 1983. During 1984, Dr. Ward stepped down as President and Dr. Tetsunao Yamamori took leadership until 2001. This was particularly significant because Dr. Y, as he is commonly known, experienced war-torn Japan as a child and thus knew intimately the consequences of hunger.

The Development Era was from 1986 through 1993 when development became the primary focus with 70% of FHI's efforts related to development by 1993. During this time, funding was broadened substantially from US and Japan to NO's in Canada, Korea, Norway, Sweden, Switzerland, and the United Kingdom. International staff grew to more than 1,600 persons spanning 26 different nationalities. Ninety percent of all staff members worked within the country of their birth. Missionaries, known as Hungry Corps (HC) staff, were raising their own support and gaining unprecedented field experience around the world. I started working with FHI during this time and was fascinated with holistic development being done. Staff positions started to define two areas of FHI: relief and development. Relief with rehabilitation included commodities, emergency health response, food security, and child assistance. Development included agriculture, church partnerships, education, child development, food production, forestry, health care, income generation, and water resource development. Along with both of these, advocacy and information, management, and information technology was developed. Symbiotic ministry was emphasized which is known today as holistic ministry.

At the beginning of the Biblical Identity Refined era, Vision of Community (VoC) was discussed in 1993 and refined through 2000. During this time, Randy Hoag, then FHI President, was influential, among others, in developing VoC. In brief, VoC is how the kingdom of God should look when FHI has completed work in a respective community. God has reconciled everything in it…to see families, churches, and leaders in the community functioning as God intends. In 1993, the corporate identity was designed which shaped the VoC impact statement and directed all activity for the entire FHI organization. The Biblical Identity Refined became the overall vision statement of FHI.

The 2001 era started with Randy Hoag taking over as President. Randy had begun work with FHI as a Hunger Corp staff during 1983 in Bolivia. From 1987 to 1991 Randy was promoted to Bolivian Country Director. For the next ten years Randy, a CPA, held many administrative positions within FHI, eventually rising through the ranks to become President in March 2001. Randy began to direct FHI from new headquarters in Bangkok, Thailand as of Fall 2003. His contribution was focused into a more people-driven organization. Empowerment of staff and human development was then top priority.

Characteristic Periods of Development in Agency & Personnel

The above case study will serve as an example of how mission agencies and personnel might proceed through periods of formation and perhaps transformation. No maturing successful agency or staff is static but will change in a dynamic process of being pro-active. This might be seen as operating in a pre-emptive manner with planning, vision, and implementation. When an agency or staff becomes or succumbs to a re-active role, survival and self-maintenance usually is the beginning of the end.

Trends in development will be discussed in each period through which agency and personnel might be progressing. The FH case study could be observed as typical. Agencies and individuals might determine what period they are currently in and then establish future plans. Periods of development work follow.

Characteristic Periods of Development	
I	Relief Emphasized
II	Development Emphasized
III	Development & Relief Balanced
IV	Biblical Identity Refined
V	Member Care & Pastoral Growth
VI	Decentralization of Ownership
VII	Spawning of New Specializations

I. Relief Emphasized

The relief period is usually what has prompted the agency group or individual (outsiders) to start action, as they see an immediate need in a community (insiders) and try to respond. That need is usually dramatic, life threatening, and requires immediate assistance. Suffering is observed on a large scale in which emotion drives a response. A definition of relief used by World Vision is "relief is the urgent provision of resources to reduce suffering resulting from a natural or man-made disaster" (Millham, 1989, 257). Emergency aid is needed quickly but will be temporary and pro-longed only when self-reliance is impossible. Development is not considered until immediate needs are met. Good relief work will transition into development work. Once a people group (insiders) can be relieved of meeting daily needs, they normally desire to become self-sufficient. Good development must teach them how to take ownership and be responsible for themselves. The Distinctives outlined later in this chapter can be used to continue this process.

II. Development Emphasized

When development is emphasized it is usually done as a reaction to a group of people's (insiders) ability to exist beyond just survival, allowing them to take responsibility for their own destiny. A need for people to be empowered is discovered. Development allows those who have been dependent to become independent. A natural direction for the community development worker (outsider) is to assist people to become independent. Thus, development arises out of common sense and need.

Dr. Deborah Ajulu, Professor and Dean of Kumi (Christian) University in northern Uganda, provides a detailed case study "Development Agencies and Holistic Empowerment" in her book *Holism in Development* (Ajulu, 2001:167-206). Out of eight agencies included in her study, four were Christian (Tearfund, World Vision UK, Emmanuel International, and Y-Care International) and four secular (Oxfam, ActionAid, ACORD, and APT Design and Development). Ajulu draws five conclusions relevant to development: (Ajulu, 2001:203-204).

1. No agency can achieve holistic empowerment on its own.

70

2. Each agency will exhibit wide differences, strengths and weaknesses, in areas of operations so that coordination of agencies is needed.

3. A new approach to project process appears—changing from blueprint approach to the development of people.

4. Powerlessness to alleviate poverty should concern the poor and the rich and powerful but normally agencies are only concerned with the poor.

5. Empowerment is recognized as a means of tackling poverty at its roots.

III. Development and Relief Balanced

While long-term development is being implemented, short-term relief is still available so assurance can be provided against returning to the emergency state of meeting basic needs. Malcolm McGregor, former International Director of SIM, makes a case for long-term and short-term missionaries when he states, "I explained that people in this generation make long term decisions in short bits. They are not less committed, but they constantly evaluate what they are do-ing. [Speaking of Jesus and the apostles] I believe they had a long-term passion and a short-term plan" (*Serving in Mission Together*, 2004:2). The editor of *Serving in Mission Together*, Carol Wilson, adds a further thought, "But whatever the season and location, the goal is always the harvest: a growing, reproducing church" (*Serving in Mission Together*, 2004:2). In essence, relief short-term workers will be needed at times and other times long-term workers who will assist in development are needed. On occasion, both are needed.

IV. Biblical Identity Refined

As an agency or a person starts to take personal account of the activity in which they are most effective, they should begin to con-centrate on areas for which they are best suited. In the case of Food for the Hungry, it was recognized that, "Besides God, FHI's most important resource is its staff. Our programs and activities will only be as effective as the staff that manage and operate them. Our work will be fundamentally flawed if we don't have the right people" (Wheeler, 2003:145). This led to development and refinement of the

Vision of Community and Corporate Identity Manual that emphasized commitment to maturity, ministry and mission. Major discussion transpired about what a community should look like when it is functioning as God intends. A large emphasis was deciding what families, church, and community leaders would be doing when VoC was functioning well. Appropriate people to meet the vision statement drove FHI to the next phase: member care and pastoral growth of staff.

V. Member Care and Pastoral Growth

The availability of pastoral and ministry resources for staff has definitely come of age. It is now common to see Human Resources Departments in mission agencies. Agency needs range from member care to educational desires. Member care is "the ongoing investment of resources by mission agencies, churches, and other mission organizations for the nurture and development of missionary personnel. It focuses on everyone in missions (missionaries, support staff, children, and families) and does so over the course of the missionary life cycle, from recruitment through retirement" (O'Donnell, 2002:4). Educational approaches are needed for staff who are varied in job responsibility, located in various parts of the world, and have few resources at their disposal. At the conclusion of a seminar on distance learning and leadership and to show need for distance education, Elliston states, "We must recognize that the Church has a greater need for leaders than we can currently meet with our present programs" (Elliston, 1997:57).

Pastoral and other community development workers can currently complete significant learning and whole degree programs at home or while overseas. Elliston states three modes of education for us to consider: formal, nonformal and informal education (Elliston, 1989:237; Elliston, 1997:13-15). **Formal programs** are associated with schools and universities that aim at certificates, diplomas, and degrees. As an example, Hope International University has been providing distance education in international development with MBA/MSM degrees and certificates since the first online course I taught in August of 1996. See website: www.hiu.edu. As another example, in 2019, I developed the Doctor of Ministry degree program for

Myitkyina Christian Seminary in Northern Myanmar. Along with other professors, I taught face-to-face courses there. **Nonformal (NFE) programs** provide planned learning outside school contexts like seminars, conferences, and internship models. NFE is currently used in many mission agencies such as Serving in Missions (SIM), "Hope for AID's," (*Serving in Mission Together*, 2004:7) and the United States Center for World Missions (USCWM) "Perspectives" classes, and Operational World-View curriculum (*Mission Frontiers*, 2004:8). Another example is a group of Bible teachers, including myself, traveling to Ghana to teach in the Christian Leadership Training Institute. See website: www.cltigh.org. **Informal programs** are less structured, may be unplanned, and used unrehearsed. Much personal counseling, personal ministry, and encouragement takes place when pastors and other leaders visit field sites. An increase in this mode of education is encouraging as it is being used more and more during this phase of development. As an example, I have traveled to Battambang, Cambodia, to teach a week-long course at the Leadership Training Institute. It is sponsored by the Cambodian Christian Churches Organization (CCCO). See website: www.hopeforcambodia.org

VI. Decentralization of Ownership

If true capacity building for management of sustainable holistic development is to take place, focus must be on the field—village and community—level. A strong case can be made for capacity building of locals and nationals when sustainable holistic development is targeted because outsiders cannot continue a work when they are not allowed in a country. Inherent in the definition of sustainability is my focus in Chapter Three: "sustainability cannot be achieved unless capacity building of national staff within their respective communities is attained. People must take precedent over programs" (Rabe, 2002:56). When leadership is centralized in main offices it can be out of touch with field needs.

In June of 2003, Food for the Hungry International initiated a move of their headquarters from Scottsdale, Arizona to Bangkok, Thailand. A major reason for such drastic move, after some thirty years in Arizona, was they wanted to be closer to their work—much of which is focused in Southeast Asia and Sub-Sahara Africa. At this time, there had already developed a long list of what FHI calls "National Organizations" or NO's. They are autonomous organizations that provide funding, commodities and staff for FHI programs. They consist of organizations in Canada, Costa Rica, Hong Kong, Japan, Korea, Norway, Sweden, Switzerland, the U.K. and the U.S.A" (Wheeler 2003:11). Decentralization had taken place, in many ways, long before 2003.

With decentralization comes partnerships with local communities. This ownership is essential for public private partnerships (PPP's) to develop with crucial stakeholders. "Partnerships between stakeholders are crucial for capacity building if sustainability is to occur as sustainability can only be accomplished if local personnel is involved" (Rabe, 2002:57). There is usually a common agreement from the beginning that local people (insiders) know better their community needs than anyone coming from outside the community (outsiders).

VII. Spawning of New Specializations

In his book *Penetrating Missions' Final Frontier*, Tetsunao Yamamori cities four qualifications for God's special envoys, as he calls the creative personnel who focus on special needs and special people groups. **First,** training must be widely available to attract a broad base including college students, midcareer candidates, and others from all over the world. **Second**, this training needs to be interesting and challenging enough to attract successful people who are bright and well educated. **Third**, training must strengthen a skill that is relevant and necessary to the 'people group' where the envoy will serve. **Fourth**, the training needs to be built on an unquestionably sound biblical base so candidates will be comfortable with it (Yamamori, 1993:68-69).

In the case of Food for the Hungry, it was a natural to allow specialty groups to break away from the original FHI mission. Some ministries might find this freedom rare and would see it as they should be guarding their "turf." When FHI began observing creative approaches to meet physical and spiritual needs of people groups, such ideas germinated into action. Therefore, Dr. Russ Mask, FHI staff, worked with FHI micro-enterprise in the Philippines and in Kenya and Uganda. Initially, the program was a loan start-up group called Faulu (Swahili meaning successful or to flourish). After working with small business savings and loan groups, it was decided a multiplication of such ideas was needed and people were essential to be trained to foster such activity. This is when Dr. Mask started work with Chalmers Institute for Economic Development, a growing arm of Covenant College in Tennessee. By allowing Dr Mask to be seconded to Chalmers, FHI was starting a new specialized group.

Another such break off is in the making after two decades of discussing symbiotic ministry, now known as holistic ministry, a whole arm of FHI developed titled Wholistic Ministry Resources. Part of this came about because of a relationship between Bob Moffitt, Founder and Director of Harvest Ministries in Phoenix, who had worked at FHI, and his predecessor, Darrow Miller, who became VP of Wholistic Ministry Resources. This idea of focus on wholistic ministry started Samaritan Strategies ministry which turned into Harvest Foundation and serves the churches all over the world today with creative holistic ministry training. Disciple Nations Alliance was also a spin off (see www.disciplenations.org).

If a boy off the farm from Central Illinois can be used in worldwide places, it is possible for anyone. In my life, I could never have imagined the spin-off God has directed over many years. From that first community outreach to homes around the local church in Salt Lake City, Utah, in 1970, to developing and teaching in the first Doctor of Ministry program in northern Myanmar starting in 2019 in Myitkyina Christian Seminary. In between, it has been a blessing and wonder to watch God send my family to Haiti, use us with neighbors, engage with students, serve in church activities, create biblical refinement formally and informally, and rub shoulders with God's leaders at various universities. In my skill area, God directed me to teach many local and international students worldwide, start and teach in a vibrant online local church Bible institute, and closely minister with a Christian seminary half-way around the world in an unreached, now reached, people group. Community development can start small, grow over years and progress into a worldwide mission outreach.

Progressive Characteristics of Development Work in Mission

When communities, groups, and individuals are advancing towards God's perspective and desire for His Kingdom, certain key elements can be observed. Not every key element is necessary for success, but the more the essential ones are used, the better chance for true accomplishment. As people grow in their understanding of God and in their actions, they will increasingly show growth in each of these distinctives.

Essential Distinctives

Listed below are key elements with examples of the expected growth for the successful Christian community developer. These might be used as indicators to determine progress.

1. **Bathe the process in prayer**. (1 Thess. 5:17) *"pray without ceasing."* Growth Example: People will stop praying routine repetitions—they will move to heart-felt requests, thanksgiving, and specific praises.

2. **Demonstrate God's love as well as tell it**. (James 2:17) *"Even so faith, if it has not works, is dead, being by itself."* Growth Example: As individuals grow, they will still talk of how God is blessing, but they will ALSO be more focused on doing, such as giving money, helping others with food, and participating in manual labor projects.

3. **Servant-leadership is shown**. (Matt. 20:28) *"...the son of man did not come to be served but to serve..."* Growth Example: Serving others becomes a high priority along with giving of time, effort, and serving the poor and needy.

4. **Spiritual relationship (priesthood) of believers is practiced.** (1 Peter 2:9 NIV) *"But you are a chosen race, a royal priesthood..."* Growth Example: Everything done by a growing believer will reflect God's love in their heart. Activity shows credit to HIM rather than credit to ourselves.

5. **Holistic ministry is taught.** (Luke 2:52) *"And Jesus kept increasing in wisdom and stature and in favor with God and men."* Growth Example: Our thinking and behavior will increasingly focus on all areas of life, including mental, physical, spiritual and social needs, not just one area.

6. **Community ownership is established.** (Acts 2:45) *"and they began selling their property and possessions, and were sharing them with all as anyone might have need."* Growth Example: We will expand horizontal relationships with people and vertical relationships with God. We tend to give up our rights and do what is best for the community or group.

7. **Participatory methods of teaching are used.** (1 Peter 5:3 NIV) *"not lording it over those entrusted to you, ..."* Growth Example: Learning increases by doing as opposed to just telling (lecturing). A partnership grows when community ownership becomes stronger for the insider.

8. **Community provides local resources for use in projects.** (Matt. 14:17 NIV) *"...We have here only five loaves of bread and two fish ..."* Growth Example: The community (insiders) will provide skills, talents and material goods more frequently, before outsiders offer their expertise and resources.

9. **Community committee is responsible with outside consultation.** (Proverbs 11:14 NIV) *"...many advisors make victory sure."* Growth Example: A representative group of insiders often become the authority for decision making—outsiders are consulted only as needed.

10. **Spiritual instruction is key component.** (Luke 8:8) *"And other seed fell into the good soil, and grew up, and produced a crop a hundred times as great. ..."* Growth Example: People needing answers to questions in their lives will increasingly seek guidance from the Bible. People will also seek God's ways through prayer and consultation with others.

Additional Distinctives

The following principles are helpful in generating growth of transformational Christian Development:

1. **Start with small programs and let them grow naturally and slowly.** (1 Cor. 3:6) *"I planted, Apollos watered, but God was causing the growth."* Growth Example: People will be more and more patient waiting on God to bless small projects. They will increasingly see God's part, their part, and outsiders' part in community development.

2. **Develop collaboration and networking with partners who can fulfill missing expertise and resources.** (1 Cor. 12:14) *"For the body is not one member, but many."* Growth Example: An openness will progressively come about to know and use skills and abilities of insiders, outsiders, and community people in and outside the church.

3. **Establish a system of measurement and accountability at the beginning**. (Nehemiah 2:5) *"...send me...that I may rebuild it."* Growth Example: Plans are made before starting so everyone knows the goal and indicators that will be evident over time.

4. **Select staff that are Christians and provide training to develop expertise**. (Philippians 2:2) *"...being of the same mind..."* Growth Example: As special areas of expertise are needed, select people with a transformed heart and life who can then learn the expertise.

5. **Staff project with people of diverse skills and interest but common goal**. (1 Cor. 12:12 NIV) *"The body is a unit, though it is made up of many parts; and though all its parts are many, they form one body..."* Growth Example: People have diverse skills and abilities BUT all should have same goals.

6. **Emphasize prevention of disease and health promotion.** (3 John 1:2) *"...be in good health..."* Growth Examples: For best long-term life, we need to take care of ourselves physically, spiritually, mentally, and socially. This honors God.

7. **Measure results in terms of multiplication, not addition.** (John 14:12) *"...greater works than these shall he do..."* Growth Example: When evaluating results, the best is to see growth compounded geometrically rather than simply adding results in a linear method.

8. **Demonstration projects should be developed and shared.** (Nehemiah 2:17 NIV) *"...you see the trouble we are in..."* Growth Example: Seeing success builds eagerness and excitement and is best for further learning.

9. **Training takes place through home visits**. (Acts 2:46) *"...breaking bread from house to house..."* Growth Examples: The best place for life teaching and learning is where one lives.

10. **A champion is needed to spearhead the vision.** (Nehemiah 2:5) "...*send me to Judah, to the city of my father's tombs...*" Growth Example: Projects need one focused person to take authority, give guidance, and rely upon for overall understanding as well as direct activity.

Concluding Remarks

Growth of development work is generally related to increased spiritual maturity. As development work progresses so does the spiritual maturity of agencies and personnel. One could assume that the increase of development work during the past three decades would have enhanced the worldwide spread of the gospel. To prove this, new comparisons and measures must be made. Reports based on information available in places like economy (e.g. Human Development Index, public debt/person, and income/person), leadership training, needs in countries and people groups, mission vision, effects of war, tyranny, and government incompetence, all assist in evaluation and analysis of the impact of development (Johnstone, 2001, *Operation World*—See www.operationworld.org).

Building the Kingdom of God in the nations is about God and who He is! Whatever period of development one is in does not matter to God. He can use anyone, at any time, in any place, no matter what stage in life they are. In fact, He desires to do that. Is more money, more people, more resources, and more agencies the answer? Perhaps we need a bigger picture of God and He will give us a bigger picture of transformation in community development.

Will we seek God, depend upon Him, search His Word, depend on Him for transformation in families, leaders and churches? Do we see His bride, the church, as Christ does? The Bible states, "... *as Christ loved the church and gave himself up for her to make her holy, cleansing her by the washing with water through the word, and to present her to himself as a radiant church, without stain or wrinkle or any other blemish, but holy and blameless*" (Ephesians 5:25-27, NIV). Our decisions matter to God, and ultimately to us, but do not change His mission and God's eventual overcoming of the world.

SUMMARY

Sharing the gospel and working with people who have physical and spiritual needs has always been a balance, even when Jesus went throughout the towns and villages. Development has become common work throughout the world, as poverty illustrates existing needs. How development is currently implemented and practiced in future Christian ministries vary. Christian ministry agencies and development workers go through a growth process that can be observed and reviewed. A contemporary view of development and respective stages can help us understand where we have been and sheds light on where we are headed. The review and analysis of characteristic periods of development can assist us to plan for needs and provide understanding of expectations in the future. Analysis of growth in distinctives necessary for successful Christian development will help us aim more precisely as we implement the community development process.

5

GIVING GENEROUSLY

You cannot serve both God and money
Matthew 6:24 (NIV, ESV)

Introduction

Giving is a natural outgrowth of a person with a transformed heart. Furthermore, most Christian agencies will reflect a transformed heart, as the agency leaders set an example. On an individual basis, giving is an outward behavior that reflects the inward heart. Paul speaks of the spiritual gifts administered to believers and with giving cites that "… *if it is contributing to the needs of others, let him give generously…*" (Romans 12:8, NIV). The word "contributing" (NIV) or "giving" (NLT) in the Greek understanding would mean "share" and often refers to sharing money. It implies those who have give to those who have not. "Generosity," which Paul uses here, is another Greek word that signifies "sincerity," because it implies goodwill.

Giving or sharing money to relieve needs is a spiritual gift but also a symbol of being a follower of the Lord Jesus Christ. Giving, as with other spiritual gifts, is administered by God to Christians but must be sustained through practice. We all are learners as we become a disciple of Jesus. As Christians, the first thing we must learn about money is that money is not ours, but it is God's. God provides us an opportunity to use money, manage it, and ultimately to reflect His heart through it, but money is still His. We are but "stewards" of His resources (1 Chron. 29:11,14).

As Christians grow in God's service, we see the needs of those around us. Paul sees the poverty of the poor in Jerusalem and provides financial help by "*this ministry to the saints*" (2 Cor. 9:1). When we see pain, it should be a joy to help abundantly. The Corinthian church sets an example, "*…they first gave themselves to the Lord and to us by the will of God*" (2 Cor. 8:5). Giving serves to advance the kingdom of God.

Jesus tells a parable of a servant who does not invest his talent well. Jesus calls him a wicked, lazy slave (Matt. 25:26). Giving randomly without wisdom is not a Christian characteristic. When giving in God's economy and directive, we should give big-heartedly so the giving will create thanksgiving, glorify God, and show generosity (2 Cor. 9:6, 8, 11, 13). When giving, we should tithe until we have acquired the habit, but then truly give as if everything we have is actually God's. Then there is no limit on giving!

Giving as an individual is the beginning of giving as a group, one community to another community. Giving as a community—church, mission agency, non-government organization, or private group of entrepreneurs—reflects the hearts of those individual leaders in the respective community. Groups will give through development, development assistance, development aid, humanitarian aid, and humanitarian assistance. These may all sound like the same thing, but in a technical sense, they produce different focus, meet different needs, and follow with different corresponding activities. All might be considered humanitarian aid, although some people would view them differently. This chapter will focus on humanitarian aid or assistance given in development settings from typically Christian groups, be they individuals, agencies, churches, or others.

Much is said about the Good Samaritan who in Luke 10:25-37 sets a standard for assisting those in need. Views of the wounded man are a collection of perspectives viewed through different lens and with individual attitudes through the eyes of the beholder:

Different Lens	Views About The Wounded Man
Law expert	he [wounded man] was a subject to discuss
Robbers	he was someone to use and exploit
Religious men	he was a problem to avoid
Innkeeper	he was a customer to serve for a fee
Samaritan	he was a human being worth caring for
Jesus	he, she, they, and we were worth dying for

When confronted with the needs of others, various attitudes and responses are generated. Jesus clearly states which attitude is acceptable to Him. With introspection, we may find ourselves responding as any of the players in the story. We need to learn afresh who our neighbors are and how best to respond to them. The outsider looks at taking action on situations with a different perspective than the person in need (insider) who is part of the existing circumstances. Doing God's will does not guarantee a comfortable life (Job 2:10; Luke 2:3-6). Sharing is exemplary as in the early church (Acts 2:44) when the believers sold possessions and goods so needs (not desires or wants) were met. Helping others is a priority as the need is noticed (Luke 13:15-16; Galatians 6:1-3) as demonstrated acts of love (John 13:35) characteristic of Christians.

Definitions

Because of differing needs and thus differing actions to meet such needs, it is important to understand the definition of key terms in community development and humanitarian aid. The following definitions will assist in understanding the focus and function within key terms.

Development—Several perspectives exist, but Myers presents a definition with a Biblical base. "Transformational development" reflects "positive change in the whole of human life materially, socially, and spiritually," based upon lifelong choices (Myers, 1999:3).

Development assistance—Long term strategy to prevent problems, like violence, consisting of external resources to reconstruct a neighborhood or country's infrastructure, institutions, rule of law, government and services, and economy towards local capacity building so a region can function independently of aid (Branczik, 2004:2).

Humanitarian aid—Such aid "is material and logistic assistance to people who need the help. It is usually short-term help until the long-term help by government and other institutions replaces it. Among the people in need are the homeless, refugees, and victims of natural disasters, wars, and famines. The primary objective of humanitarian aid is to save lives, alleviate suffering, and maintain human dignity." [http://en.m.wikipedia.org/wiki/Humanitarian_aid].

In the immediate area of conflict, the primary aim is preventing human casualties and ensuring access to the basics for survival: water, sanitation, food, shelter, and health care. Apart from the main fighting, the priority is to assist people who have been displaced, prevent spread of conflict, support relief work, and prepare for rehabilitation (www.beyondintractability.org/essay/humanitarian_aid/).

Development aid—Essentially, the same as humanitarian aid with additional focus on addressing the underlying socioeconomic factors which may have fostered the crisis. "Development aid (also development assistance, international aid, overseas aid or foreign aid) is aid given by the developed countries (the "haves") for sustainable development in the developing countries (the "have nots"). It is distinguished from humanitarian aid, being aimed at alleviating poverty in the long term" (Firoz, 2005:1).

Humanitarian assistance—Usually it is common to interchange this with humanitarian aid. Although some might call humanitarian assistance more long-term directed towards peace building in violent conflict (Barbolet, 2006, 1).

Goals of Development and Humanitarian Assistance

There are many reasons why development and humanitarian assistance are provided. Various reasons for giving include guilt or obligation, donating for personal reasons, providing charity, meeting needs, helping people, and building relationships. Additional reasons are presenting a bribe, investing in the future, peace offerings, paying for recompense, granting from wealth, being generous and benevolent, and forming a legacy, etc. Some reasons are good all the time and some are good much of the time and some are not good anytime. Most depend upon the circumstance of the beneficiary and the heart of the donor. The goals of the recipient and the donor make the difference.

International Alert states a "conflict-sensitive development" (i.e. any area needing aid because of conflict, normally military intervention) is complex and such areas affected by war cause serious planning and implementation as the result can be disastrous (Barbolet, 2006:2). They state the following goals should be worked towards:
- Research with partners—work together towards mutual goals
- Global-level research on more effective responses—search to confirm action

- Advocating—build partnership and collaboration
- Bringing—consistently improving holistic life
- Providing—setting the example and encouragement

Among the hundreds of humanitarian agencies, including Christian and non-Christian, perhaps the largest organization with the greatest access is the National American Red Cross. Being on the boards of various local Red Cross Chapters, including Orange County Red Cross in Santa Ana, California, I will make some observations. The goals cited in response to humanitarian assistance (i.e. those foreigners giving from **outside** the community working with those who normally live and exist **inside** the community) are:

- Simple low-cost intervention—keep costs within reach of community
- Mobilize and empower communities—build local ownership
- Broker partnerships—collaboration with helpful partners
- Build local capacities—connect community with their resources
- Greater and broader focus for greater impact—set vision high

In a presentation at the Orange County Red Cross headquarters on October 25, 2006, titled, "Red Cross International Humanitarian Assistance," Apurva Patel, Director of Partnership & Program Development in International Services of Red Cross, cited key areas of involvement in humanitarian assistance as:

1. *Community Health and Disease Control*—Examples include measles immunization initiative launched in February 2001 in over 40 African countries—$1 per child www.measlesinitiative.org in partnership with WHO, CDC, UNICEF, UN Foundation as well as Malaria Initiative where $10 per child provides a bed net, education, and follow-up.

2. *Community Restoration and Rebuilding*—Examples include training, educational and community-oriented programs and events like the 23rd Annual Disaster Academy for emergency response professionals in Santa Ana, CA, Super CPR Sunday at Angel Stadium with over 1000 participants (see www.oc-redcross.org), and building emergency hospitals in various parts of the world. A further

example is the "Riders for Hope" in Kenya where medication is delivered to villages on bicycles.

3. *Disaster Preparedness*—Examples include home fire responses (e.g. Sierra wildfires in CA), Katrina, Rita, and Wilma hurricanes, and health and safety classes taught. Over the next three years, the Red Cross Tsunami Recovery Program planned to construct 1000 wells to benefit over 19,000 people in Sri Lanka. Along with this, Sri Lanka's local Red Cross Society plans to teach community members about proper hygiene and sanitation practices. Since the tsunami occurred, the American Red Cross, working with partners in the International Red Cross and Red Crescent Movement and other humanitarian organizations, has helped more than 38 million people in tsunami-affected countries. See website www.redcross.org for more information.

Of course, many other types of humanitarian assistance are provided worldwide by the Red Cross Society and Red Crescent Movements, including such things as service to military families, communication for disaster family members, HIV prevention messages to more than 750,000 youth in Guyana, Haiti, and Tanzania, and assisting as well as teaching in International Humanitarian Law (IHL). The American Red Cross, alone, is part of the world's largest humanitarian movement with a network of more than 185 Red Cross and Red Crescent Societies and approximately 97 million members and volunteers. Global health initiatives focus on reducing child mortality, improving material health, and combating infectious diseases.

Church, missionary, and community development personnel can learn much from observing what is going on around them. Even though some may be upset that government and non-governmental organizations (NGOs) have taken over previously considered ministries of the church, there is a new breed of workers who are penetrating missions' final frontier. Tetsunao Yamamori, former President of Food for the Hungry International, a Christian relief & development agency meeting physical and spiritual needs worldwide, writes about this new strategy for unreached peoples in his book titled, *Penetrating Missions' Final Frontier*. He states in his preface that:

The specific focus of this strategy [effectively evange-lizing the thousands of people groups] is the unreached peoples that share both of the two most basic human needs. These are the *physical* need of adequate food, clean water and reasonable health, and the *spiritual* need for salvation through Jesus Christ (Yamamori, 1993:13).

In many ways, it is not that common church ministries are being consumed by government and NGO agencies, but instead, it is that the church is surrendering its responsibility by default. Goals of the church are still what Jesus stated in His departing command:

> *Therefore go and make disciples of all nations, bap-tizing them in the name of the Father and of the Son and of the Holy Spirit, and teaching them to obey everything I have commanded you. And surely I am with you always, to the very end of the age* (Matthew 28:19 20, NIV, 1984).

The goals of Jesus truly must be the goals of the church. Per-haps it is up to the church to review Jesus' methods as outlined in various accounts of his ministry: *Jesus went through all the towns and villages, teaching in their synagogues, preaching the good news of the kingdom and healing every disease and sickness* (Matthew 9:35 NIV) and as He suggested His servant "*...gives even a cup of cold water...*" (Matthew 10:42, NIV). In our beginning example of The Good Samaritan we find Jesus makes this mandate:

1. **The Great Commandment**—Answering what must be done to inherit eternal life the expert in the law responds, "*He answered: 'Love the Lord your God with all your heart and with all your soul and with all your strength and with all your mind'; and, 'Love your neighbor as yourself.'*" "*You have answered correctly,*" Jesus re-plied. "*Do this, and you will live*" (Luke 10:27-28 NIV).

2. **The Great Commission**—Jesus asked the expert in the law, "*Which of these three do you think was a neighbor to the man who fell into the hands of robbers?*" The expert in the law replied, "*The one who had mercy on him.*" Jesus told him, "*Go and do likewise*" (Luke 10:36-37 NIV).

Biblical Standard for Giving Aid

Humanitarian aid is commonly delivered by governmental and non-governmental aid organizations, including the church and other Christian groups. Most such agencies are funded by donations from individuals, corporations, governments, and other organizations. The funding and delivery of humanitarian aid is increasingly being organized at a city, regional, or international level to facilitate faster and more effective responses to major emergencies affecting large numbers of people. Denomination headquarters are also sometimes the umbrella by which individual church groups distribute aid.

Before we look at how Christian groups should distribute aid, it is insightful to learn how Beyond Intractability, known as "A Free Knowledge Base on More Constructive Approaches to Destructive Conflict," states who does it. They say the four main actors in humanitarian aid and development assistance are:

- International (IOs) and Regional Organizations (ROs):
- Unilateral Assistance:
- Non-Governmental Organizations (NGOs):
- Military (Branczik, 2004:2).

From this summary we might see the church fitting into an IO, RO or NGO category. In this light, the giving of aid has at least four key principles that must be addressed in order to meet Biblical standards: The attitude of the giver, sacrifice and value of the gift, the proportional amount provided by the donor, and general Scriptural principles that should be followed when giving. Below are Biblical references (NIV) that demonstrate the four Christian principles for giving.

Attitude of the Giver Must Be True

1. God senses a true heart through what and how we give. *In the course of time Cain brought some of the fruits of the soil as an offering to the Lord. But Abel brought fat portions from some of his firstborn of his flock. The Lord looked with favor on Abel and his offering, but on Cain and his offering he did not look with favor. So Cain was very angry, and his face was downcast* (Gen. 4:3-5).

2. A relationship of giving generously as a commitment to God

is our focus. *Then the whole Israelite community withdrew from Moses' presence, and everyone who was willing and whose heart moved him came and brought an offering to the Lord for the work on the Tent of Meeting, for all its service, and for the sacred garments* (Exodus 35:20-21).

3. Giving should be cheerful and not reluctantly. *Moses said to the whole Israelite community, "This is what the Lord has commanded: From what you have, take an offering for the Lord. Everyone who is willing is to bring to the Lord an offering of gold, silver and bronze;* (Ex. 35:4-5).

The entire tithe of the herd and flock—every tenth animal that passes under the shepherd's rod—will be holy to the Lord. He must not pick out the good from the bad or make any substitution... (Lev. 27:32-33).

Each man should give what he has decided in his heart to give, not reluctantly or under compulsion, for God loves a cheerful giver (2 Cor. 9:7).

4. Personal Investment is Made. In helping his son Solomon prepare for building the temple, King David states, *Besides, in my devotion to the temple of my God I now give my personal treasures of gold and silver for the temple of my God, over and above everything I have provided...* (1Chron. 29:3).

5. We give based upon our abilities. After hearing of a severe famine in Judea, *The disciples, each according to his ability, decided to provide help for the brothers living in Judea* (Acts 11:29).

6. Our real priorities are shown. *Do not sacrifice to the Lord your God an ox or a sheep that has any defect or flaw in it, for that would be detestable to him* (Deut. 17:1).

7. Ask if my convictions keep me from helping others. Jesus in the synagogue observes, *...and a man with a shriveled hand was there. Looking for a reason to accuse Jesus, they asked him, "Is it lawful to heal on the Sabbath?" He said to them, "If any of you has*

a sheep and it falls into a pit on the Sabbath, will you not take hold of it and lift it out? How much more valuable is a man than a sheep! Therefore it is lawful to do good on the Sabbath" (Matt. 12:10-12).

8. Giving to get something in return is not acceptable. *But when you give to the needy, do not let your left hand know what your right hand is doing, so that your giving may be in secret...* (Matt. 6:3-4).

9. Your heart should care for those who are afflicted. *As you know, it was because of an illness that I first preached the gospel to you. Even though my illness was a trial to you, you did not treat me with contempt or scorn. Instead, you welcomed me as if I were an angel of God, as if I were Christ Jesus himself* (Gal. 4:13-14).

10. Follow Jesus who sets our example by showing a caring nature. *When Jesus saw her weeping, and the Jews who had come along with her also weeping, he was deeply moved in spirit and troubled. "Where have you laid him?" he asked. "Come and see, Lord," they replied. Jesus wept. Then the Jews said, "See how he loved him!" But some of them said, "Could not he who opened the eyes of the blind man have kept this man from dying?" Jesus, once more deeply moved, came to the tomb. It was a cave with a stone laid across the entrance* (John 11:33-38).

11. Confirm there is an internal spirit of giving. *Woe to you, teachers of the law and Pharisees, you hypocrites! You give a tenth of your spices—mint, dill and cummin. But you have neglected the more important matters of the law—justice, mercy and faithfulness. You should have practiced the latter, without neglecting the former. You blind guides! You strain out a gnat but swallow a camel* (Matt. 23:23-24).

The men of Nineveh will stand up at the judgment with this generation and condemn it; for they repented at the preaching of Jonah, and now one greater than Jonah is here. The Queen of the South will rise at the judgment with this generation and condemn it; for she came from the ends of the earth to listen to Solomon's wisdom, and now one greater than Solomon is here. "When an evil spirit comes out of a man, it goes through arid places seeking rest and does not find it. Then it says, 'I will return to the house I left.' When it arrives, it finds the house unoccupied, swept clean and put in order (Matt. 12:41-44).

12. We should have a generous and gracious heart that sincerely reflects our love. *But just as you excel in everything—in faith, in speech, in knowledge, in complete earnestness and in your love for us—see that you also excel in this grace of giving. I am not commanding you, but I want to test the sincerity of your love by comparing it with the earnestness of others* (2 Cor. 8:7-8).

True Sacrifice is Giving Something of Value

1. We show how we value something by our gracious behavior. *David said to him, "Let me have the site of your threshing floor so I can build an altar to the Lord, that the plague on the people may be stopped. Sell it to me at the full price." Araunah said to David, "Take it! Let my lord the king do whatever pleases him. Look, I will give the oxen for the burnt offerings, the threshing sledges for the wood, and the wheat for the grain offering. I will give all this." But King David replied to Araunah, "No, I insist on paying the full price. I will not take for the Lord what is yours, or sacrifice a burnt offering that costs me nothing"* (1 Chron. 21:22-24).

2. There is a cost of following Jesus. *Then a teacher of the law came to him and said, "Teacher, I will follow you wherever you go." Jesus replied, "Foxes have holes and birds of the air have nests, but the Son of Man has no place to lay his head"* (Matt. 8:19-20).

Jesus answered, "If you want to be perfect, go, sell your possessions and give to the poor, and you will have treasure in heaven. Then come, follow me." When the young man heard this, he went away sad, because he had great wealth (Matt. 19:21-22).

Jesus looked at him and loved him. "One thing you lack," he said. "Go sell everything you have and give to the poor, and you will have treasure in heaven. Then come, follow me." At this the man's face fell. He went away sad, because he had great wealth (Mark 10:21-22).

3. Jesus uses whatever we have and give to meet and exceed the needs. *And he directed the people to sit down on the grass. Taking the five loaves and the two fish and looking up to heaven, he gave thanks and broke the loaves. Then he gave them to the disciples, and the disciples gave them to the people. They all ate and were satisfied, and the disciples picked up twelve basketfuls of broken pieces that were left over. The number of those who ate was about five thousand men, besides women and children* (Matt. 14:19-21).

So they gathered them and filled twelve baskets with the pieces of the five barley loaves left over by those who had eaten (John 6:13).

4. Without being requested, volunteering to meet the needs of others sets a high standard. *Some men came, bringing to him a paralytic, carried by four of them* (Mark 2:3).

5. Comfort those in pain by listening, perhaps their greatest need at the time. *Then Job replied: "I have heard many things like these; miserable comforters are you all! Will your long-winded speeches never end? What ails you that you keep on arguing? I also could speak like you, if you were in my place; ..."* (Job 16:1-4a).

Give Proportional to What You Have Been Given
1. The amount to give is determined by what God has given you. *Three times a year all your men must appear before the Lord your God at the place he will choose: at the Feast of Unleavened Bread, the Feast of Weeks and the Feast of Tabernacles. No man should appear before the Lord empty-handed: Each of you must bring a gift in proportion to the way the Lord your God has blessed you* (Deut. 16:16-17)

2. Upon receiving, give to God first and give your best. *Honor the Lord with your wealth, with the first fruits of all your crops; then your barns will be filled to overflowing, and your vats will brim over with new wine* (Prov. 3:9-10).

"A son honors his father, and a servant his master. If I am a father, where is the honor due me? If I am a master, where is the respect

due me?" says the Lord Almighty. "It is you, O priests, who show contempt for my name. But you ask, 'How have we shown contempt for your name?' You place defiled food on my altar. But you ask, 'How have we defiled you?' By saying that the Lord's table is contemptible. When you bring blind animals for sacrifice, is that not wrong? When you sacrifice crippled or diseased animals, is that not wrong? Try offering them to your governor! Would he be pleased with you? Would he accept you?" says the Lord Almighty (Mal. 1:6-8).

3. Giving a little is better than giving nothing. *Another of his disciples, Andrew, Simon Peter's brother, spoke up, "Here is a boy with five small barley loaves and two small fish, but how far will they go among so many?"* (John 6:8-9).

4. Give freely and without prodding. *When they arrived at the house of the Lord in Jerusalem, some of the heads of the families gave freewill offerings toward the rebuilding of the house of God on its site. According to their ability they gave to the treasury for this work 61,000 drachmas of gold, 5,000 minas of silver and 100 priestly garments* (Ezr. 2:68-69).

Heal the sick, raise the dead, cleanse those who have leprosy, drive out demons. Freely you have received, freely give (Matt. 10:8).

Remember this: Whoever sows sparingly will also reap sparingly, and whoever sows generously will also reap generously. Each man should give what he has decided in his heart to give, not reluctantly or under compulsion, for God loves a cheerful giver. And God is able to make all grace abound to you, so that in all things at all times, having all that you need, you will abound in every good work (2 Cor. 9:6-8).

5. Give sacrificially. *As he looked up, Jesus saw the rich putting their gifts into the temple treasury. He also saw a poor widow put in two very small copper coins. "I tell you the truth," he said, "this poor widow has put in more than all the others. All these people gave their gifts out of their wealth; but she out of her poverty put in all she had to live on"* (Luke 21:1-4).

Out of the most severe trial, their overflowing joy and their extreme poverty welled up in rich generosity. For I testify that they gave as much as they were able, and even beyond their ability. Entirely on their own, they urgently pleaded with us for the privilege of sharing in this service to the saints. And they did not do as we expected, but they gave themselves first to the Lord and then to us in keeping with God's will (2 Cor. 8:2-5).

General Scriptural Principles of Giving

1. Willingness to give liberally to the needy sets an excellent example. *And here is my advice about what is best for you in this matter: Last year you were the first not only to give but also to have the desire to do so. Now finish the work, so that your eager willingness to do it may be matched by your completion of it, according to your means. For if the willingness is there, the gift is acceptable according to what one has, not according to what he does not have.*

Our desire is not that others might be relieved while you are hard pressed, but that there might be equality. At the present time your plenty will supply what they need, so that in turn their plenty will supply what you need. Then there will be equality, as it is written: "He who gathered much did not have too much, and he who gathered little did not have too little" (2 Cor. 8:10-15).

2. To best help others we must get involved in their lives. *When Abram heard that his relative had been taken captive, he called out the 318 trained men born in his household and went in pursuit as far as Dan. During the night Abram divided his men to attack them and he routed them, pursuing them as far as Hobah, north of Damascus. He recovered all the goods and brought back his relative Lot and his possessions, together with the women and the other people* (Gen. 14:14-16).

3. Continue to work with and embrace those who accept the message of the kingdom. *When you enter a house, first say, 'Peace to this house.' If a man of peace is there, your peace will rest on him; if not, it will return to you. Stay in that house, eating and drinking whatever they give you, for the worker deserves his wages. Do not*

move around from house to house (Luke 10:5-7).

4. We should show compassion instead of judging others. *But Jesus bent down and started to write on the ground with his finger. When they kept on questioning him, he straightened up and said to them, "If any one of you is without sin, let him be the first to throw a stone at her"* (John 8:6b-7).

5. Jesus showed compassion to those in need. *He took her by the hand and said to her, "Talitha koum!" (which means, "Little girl, I say to you, get up!"). Immediately the girl stood up and walked around (she was twelve years old). At this they were completely astonished* (Mark 5:41-42).

Problems with Humanitarian Aid and Development Assistance

Great challenges exist as humanitarian aid and development assistance is distributed. The same challenges with humanitarian aid apply to development assistance but some additional ones may apply here. A pastor friend of mine tells the story of a national in Africa who told him to "stop sending us your money as it is keeping us from growing, becoming self-reliant, and from developing partnerships. Dependency is not good for us." There has always existed a divide between those seeing the plight in view from outside the situation (outsiders) with those IN the circumstances (insiders). From this example alone we can question if aid is always the correct decision.

According to Beyond Intractability (www.beyondintractability. org) there is additional rationale for withholding aid.

> The greatest challenges for humanitarian aid and development assistance are efficiency, effectiveness, and extreme complex political, economic and social side effects that are associated with them. It has become increasingly clear that aid is not a panacea. Although externally driven, humanitarian aid and development assistance programs inevitably take on roles within the conflict and in the societies in which they operate (Branczik, 2004:3).

With background and experience, International Alert has out-lined some negatives of humanitarian aid which will be discussed later in reference with examples.

> At International Alert, our original focus on develop-ment work was to understand the unintended nega-tive consequences of development and humanitarian aid projects in conflict zones. This learning has been instrumental in building an understanding of how the development sector works and of the key conflict/de-velopment issues and challenges. However, it is not enough for development agencies simply to avoid negative impacts of their work. The challenge now is to find ways for them to make a positive contribution to building peace in contexts where social tensions run high, where there is active violent conflict, and in so-called post-conflict situations (Barbolet, February 2006:1-2).

As a summary, we shall divide the problems with humanitarian aid into categories, including those mentioned by Branczik (the first three) and cite examples as additional principles. Examples of chal-lenges are given for further awareness and application.

1. Efficiency and Effectiveness—corruption, overhead, meet-ing perceived needs, greed...

2. Political Dilemmas—governmental oversight & costs, na-tional & international view...

3. Criticisms of Humanitarian Organizations—administrative costs vs. field needs, duplication...

4. Position and Personnel turnover—high turnover, personal views, professional training...

5. Increased Danger to National Staff—war zones, personal views, tribal conflict...

6. HIV/AIDS—implementation of strategies, health standards, coordination, follow-up...

7. Communication and Travel—coordination with others, du-plication, cost...

8. Competition/Corporation between Churches and NGO's—

biblical vs. government…

9. Donor Demands—donor designations, lack of all facts, emotion, personal experience…

10. Religious Beliefs and Ordinances—biblical interpretation, duplication, jealousness…

Conclusions & Recommendations

A debate exists over how to improve humanitarian aid and development assistance with reduced negative consequences, promoted quality of living and saving of lives for the beneficiaries. When we factor in Christian principles, it is even more vital as we are representing God's way to recipients and beneficiaries. That said, a few key ideas are suggested to consider when providing humanitarian aid.

1. Giving is Complex, Challenging and sometimes Dangerous. For example, U.S. foreign aid began with the Point Four Program of Harry S. Truman. His inaugural address on January 20, 1949, said, "We must embark on a bold new program for…the improvement and growth of underdeveloped areas. More than half the people of the world are living in conditions approaching misery. For the first time in history, humanity possesses the knowledge and the skill to relieve the suffering of these people" (Easterly, 2006:24).

2. Beneficiary Concerns (Donors vs. Recipients). A third-party involvement is lacking success because donors are demanding donations be used for designated areas but outsiders delivering the aid are caught when need is observed to vary from an original plan.

3. Address Corruption. "High aid revenues [especially from oil revenues] going to the national government benefit political insiders, often corrupt insiders, who will vigorously oppose democracy that would lead to more equal distribution of aid" (Easterly, 2006:135). A method of decreasing such temptation is essential, especially in countries where annual income is under $1,000 USD.

4. Reinforce the Purpose of Giving. We must review and question motives for giving. Following Biblical standards for giving will

provide some success.

5. Follow Biblical Standards for Transformation. Intentional capacity development (i.e. their ability to do something) by outsiders for insider transformation is essential for sustainability. Outsiders can set the spiritual example.

6. Identification with the People. Outsiders must work hard at building relationships with insiders to be accepted and meet expectations and needs.

7. Broaden Focus of Church Activities. Churches must go beyond giving money. Rather, they must set an example meeting all human needs in their local neighborhoods then duplicate such examples in regions beyond. Involvement of congregations with time, talent, relationships, and other resources is required.

8. Holistic Mission Essential. The total needs of people should be considered by including physical, social, mental, and spiritual well-being (Luke 2:52).

SUMMARY

Giving may seem harmless, right, and look beneficial, but can be a big mistake. When humanitarian aid is provided in community development, it must reflect concern for positive change in the whole of human life. Without such results, God is hindered and the poor are obstructed. This chapter provides an overview of humanitarian and development aid, its goals and how it should be given. It also presents the potential and real problems associated with providing aid as part of Christian community development and the views of those outside the circumstance versus those inside the circumstance. The key principles and Biblical examples, presented as a scriptural perspective, are essential to the Christian's mission. A review and possible change in philosophy and practice for providing humanitarian aid is a key responsibility for Christians who desire to promote community development that glorifies God.

EPILOGUE

The grace of the Lord Jesus be with all. Amen.
Revelation 22:21

Commentary

I will never forget a trip I took to Israel a few years ago when we traveled to Caesarea Philippi, an ancient Roman city in the Golan Heights of northern Israel. At the base of Mount Hermon, Jesus was asking his disciples, *"Who do people say that the Son of man is?"* (Matthew 16:13). The disciples gave individual answers, but Peter said, *"Thou art the Christ, the Son of the living God"* (Matthew 16:16). With that correct answer, Jesus responds by saying to Peter that a church will be built—that was the first time church is mentioned in the Bible. Peter means the little rock (Greek Petros) but Jesus is the big rock (Greek Petra) on which the church will be built. Jesus was the foundation of the church.

As we sat on some rocks nearby, we discussed the Matthew 16 Scripture and viewed one of the largest springs feeding the Jordan River. I was mesmerized with the beauty, rolling waters, and park-like view of the stream heading south. Then we were made aware of an exceptionally large opening into the mountain, probably ten feet high and ten feet wide. This was the site of the Greek god Pan who was worshiped there. This cave was believed to be the gateway to the underworld. Many sacrifices and pagan worship took place there in order to appease the gods. Still Jesus brought his disciples there, as he revealed to them, He is the Messiah. In these surroundings, Jesus announced the church to come.

This place has a long history. It is where Herod the Great built the Temple of Augustus in 19 B.C. to honor Caesar. Before the Roman era, the Greeks built many sanctuaries where they also worshiped the god Pan by throwing animal sacrifices into the bottomless pool inside the cave entrance. It was such a wicked place that many rabbis forbid good Jews from coming here. Still Jesus started His church here. Jesus set the pattern for reaching into the world of the enemy. Traditionally, this is the site of the Transfiguration of Jesus (Matthew 17:1-8) where Jesus established a foothold into the real world of the evil one.

This is the same place that Mark Twain made a stop in 1867. He described Caesarea Philippi like this: "scattered everywhere, in the paths and in the woods, are Corinthian capitals, broken porphyry pillars, and little fragments of sculpture; and up yonder in the precipice where the fountain gushes out, are well-worn Greek inscriptions over niches in the rock where in ancient times the Greeks, and after the Romans, worship the sylvan god Pan" (Land of the Bible website: www.land-of-the-bible.com/Caesarea_Philippi). This is a notable place for Jesus to tell his disciples that He is the Messiah and to establish the church in the most sinful place in Israel. As a believer, *Step Outside of Your Church, Expand Your World!*

The church is simply "people assembled" as translated from the Greek word "ekklasia." It means a called-out company, assembly or congregation of people. Never do we see in the Bible the church as a building, organization, or business. It is the people who have believed in and received Jesus and his teachings. The true church are those people who have responded to "...*the word of faith which we are preaching, that if you confess with your mouth Jesus as Lord, and believe in your heart that God raised Him from the dead, you shall be saved; for with the heart man believes, resulting in righteousness, and with the mouth he confesses, resulting in salvation*" (Romans 10:8-10).

The mission of the church is believers united with God to proclaim the gospel, the good news, to the world. This is done through **worship** and **work**. Just before Jesus ascended into heaven from the Mount of Olives, the Bible states, "*And when they saw Him, they worshiped Him...*" (Matthew 28:17). The Bible does mention key activities of the church in **worship**, "*And they [believers] were continually devoting themselves to the apostles' teaching and to fellowship, to the breaking of bread and to prayers*" (Acts 2:42).

The church has four key activities which are:
1. instructing biblical doctrine,
2. providing a place for fellowship,

3. celebrating the Lord's supper, and

4. teaching how to pray.

When Peter preached on the day of Pentecost, about 3,000 people were added and the church was born and given a purpose. Jesus tells His disciples in His last words to them before ascending to heaven, *"All authority has been given to Me in heaven and on earth. Go therefore and make disciples of all the nations, baptizing them in the name of the Father and the Son and the Holy Spirit, teaching them to observe all that I commanded you; and lo, I am with you always, even to the end of the age"* (Matthew 28:18-20). The church should **worship AND work** to "make disciples" or followers of Jesus Christ. Some would say the church must do two works: evangelism and discipleship. Others will say God's program for the church is "come and worship, go and work." Both are correct as we build the church locally and throughout the world.

Interpretation

The church function is mission outreach in this world. We believers should be going into the world sharing what we know about our Lord, the Son of the Living God. Building the local church into a strong and honorable organism is good—organisms grow, function together with many parts, maintain life, and multiply. Certainly, we should be focused **inwardly** to the church by practicing the four purposes in Acts 2:42. The body of Christ should be well respected, setting a great example and be a growing organism showing life to the world. The church should also be focused **outwardly** spawning new specialized groups (See Chapter 4, Period VII) focused upon transformation of our community and beyond to other communities worldwide. In the midst of pagan worship and ungodly practices, the church should be reaching out with the power of influence to our local neighborhood (Jerusalem), then to the region around it (Judea) and then to surrounding communities not like us (Samaria) and even worldwide (remotest part of the earth). Jesus gives such command in Acts 1:8.

When the Holy Spirit comes alive in us, we should go DO something by the power of that Spirit. Knowledge is good and some Biblical knowledge is essential BUT we need to use and apply it by

DOING something in our community of influence. Some would call this ministry. As Jesus demonstrated, we too should enter the world of people all around us. These people we influence will grow in their own unique way by the love we have shown them which they will show to others in their area of influence. The church multiples!

An Example

It is with similar such focus of the church that fifty Chinese were brought to Hope International University to study graduate business and education. In 2003 they graduated and went back to China to continue their professions. Some three years later, a group of us, including George West, Chair of the Graduate Education Department, and me, representing the Graduate Management Department, traveled to Beijing, China, to have a reunion. My poem tells about that group. I presented "The Spectacular Beijing Fifty" at the Three-Year Reunion in Beijing, China, with all but a few of the fifty in attendance.

The Spectacular Beijing Fifty
By Alan N. Rabe
Presented at the Three-Year Reunion in Beijing China
March 25, 2006

The packing, the travel, the goodbyes
All started in China with joy and many sighs.

Because life was about to change in major ways
For the Spectacular Beijing Fifty in coming days.

With everything in suitcases, and boxes as big as houses,
Goodbyes were finally said to jobs, friends, children and spouses.

The normal twelve hours aboard the plane
Had diversion to other places of fame.

This was all for very good reason
So Western names could be selected in season.

If it were not for Great Britain in the plan
London may have been named Sam, Joe or Dan.

In September 2001 the Spectacular Beijing Fifty did land
At LAX, their new home of the angels, freeways and sand.

The drive to Hope produced many new faces.
As this home was so different from China places.

Once at Hope the dorms were found to be too close
So plans were made for Nutwood Apartments by the host.

This would allow for cooking with more oil
Even though cafeteria food was good; home cooking was worth the toil.

Much new and different learning took place at Hope
While everyone, with time, learned to cope.

103

All of the faculty loved the Spectacular Beijing Fifty best
Including Drs. Henry, Price, Elliston, Mutunga, Rabe, and West.

All at Hope send their sincere love and warm greetings
Including Dr. Price with great thanks for the public policy meetings.

But it was not only the classrooms that brought good times
Dinner at West's, trips with Ben, and discussions with Alan formed minds.

For me, discussions on life, Socrates, values and the times
Caused thinking, changed ideas, built vision and established deep binds.

The year and more in the USA was tough
As staying away from family and job so long was rough.

But that great sacrifice on your parts
Molded, changed and so filled many, many hearts.

We at Hope are so very proud
As weekly we speak about you so loud.

To know of all your promotions so grand
It is now time for us to extend another hand.

We should not and cannot let this good thing end
Our hearts desire and plea is for you to select others to send.

Our request is for you to share and multiply the good given you
By sending your best to Hope so they may have success too.

Because of you, we at Hope are people who are better.
Please help us as we try to be better together.

Thank You!

BARNABAS

OBJECTIVES: By the end of this lesson, participants will:

1.   Observe how encouragement can be a forceful action to individuals and a Church.

2.   Identify how we should intercede by mentoring those needing assistance.

3.   List characteristics of a godly encourager.

4.   Describe how essential it is to disciple others and then turn leadership over to them.

INTRODUCTION

Read Acts 9:10-31 Scripture where Barnabas Intercedes for a Troublemaker. Then ask the SHOWD questions: What do you **see**? What was **happening**? Does this happen in **our** place? **Why** does it happen there? What can we **do** about it?

LESSON
I. Overview: Barnabas Intercedes for a Troublemaker (Acts 9:10-31)

A. In Acts 4:36-37 what can you tell us about Barnabas?
Answer: First mentioned in bible here, Barnabas was a Levite called Joseph. The apostles knew him. His name means Son of Encouragement (Exhortation or Consolation). He owned land, sold it to meet needs of new believers.

B. What has happened to Saul?
Answer: Saul was converted, became blind, and did not eat or drink for 3 days (vs. 9) on his way to harm Christians in Damascus (vs. 13-14).
Vs. 17 Saul is filled with the Holy Spirit and gets his sight back and was baptized.
Vs. 20 Saul immediately began to proclaim Jesus as the Son of God.

All who heard him were amazed (vs. 21).

Vs. 22 Saul was so powerful proving Jesus is the Christ that the Jews plotted to kill him (vs. 23).

His disciples let him down from a wall in the night so he could escape to go 150 miles south to Jerusalem (vs. 25-26).

C. How did the disciples respond to Saul when he came to Jerusalem? (vs. 26)
Answer: They were afraid of him and did not believe him.

D. What did Barnabas do to help Saul?
Answer: Took him to the disciples and spoke on Saul's behalf. Barnabas told of the good works Saul was doing and how he proclaimed Christ.

E. What did the disciples do with Saul?
Answer: Sent Saul to his home Tarsus, some 500 miles north.

F. How did the church respond?
Answer: (vs. 31) Church enjoyed peace, being built up, and moved on in the fear of the Lord and comfort of Holy Spirit. Church continued to increase.

II. Overview: Barnabas encourages a church and an individual (Acts 11:19-26)

A. What was happening in Antioch?
Answer: Persecution arose after Stephen's stoning and believers scattered. They only spoke God's word to the Jews. Some started to speak Jesus to the Greeks too (vs. 20) and a large number believed (vs. 21).

B. What did the disciples in Jerusalem do about the Greeks being saved (vs. 22)?
Answer: Sent Barnabas to Antioch to see what was going on.

C. What did Barnabas find happening in Antioch?

Answer: Barnabas saw the grace of God, rejoiced with them and began to encourage them to seek the Lord.

D. What characteristics did Barnabas show? What kind of man was he (vs. 24)?
Answer: He was a good man, full of Holy spirit and faith, convincing them to believe in the Lord.

E. What did Barnabas do to help the church grow?
Answer: Went to Tarsus to get Saul and brought Saul to Antioch to help teach. They both taught for one year with Barnabas discipling Saul. It was the first time the disciples were called Christians (vs. 26).

III. Overview: Barnabas turns leadership over to Paul (Acts 12:25-13:1-12)

A. What was happening in Jerusalem?
Answer: Great persecution was taking place with the disciples back in Jerusalem, but the word of God grew and multiplied.

B. What happened when Paul and Barnabas returned to Antioch form Jerusalem (vs. 12:25-13:4)?
Answer: Holy Spirit told church to "set apart" Saul and Barnabas to send them away to minister on the first missionary journey.

C. What happened when Paul and Barnabas got to Salamis (vs. 5-8)?
Answer: The preached he Word of God (vs. 5) and was asked by the governor, Sergius, to share Jesus (vs. 7). However, the magician/ sorcerer, Elymas, was opposing them and tried to keep the governor from faith in Jesus (vs. 8).

D. What did Saul, also called Paul, do to the sorcerer (vs. 9-11)?
Answer: Paul starred at him, told him he was of the devil, and to stop. The sorcerer became blind and they had to lead him around.

E. How did this affect the governor, Sergius (vs. 12)?
Answer: Sergius believed in Jesus and was amazed at the Word of God.

F. Who was the dominant leader now, Paul or Barnabas?
Answer: Paul was leading as Barnabas turned over leadership to him.

G. Rest of New Testament, Paul and Barnabas work together but Paul is main leader until a sharp dispute in Acts 15:2, 39. What happened there?
Answer: Legalism of circumcision was coming into the Antioch church. Paul and Barnabas disagreed on it and were sent to Jerusalem disciples to decide what was correct.

H. Did Paul and Barnabas ever work together again (vs. 1 Cor. 9:6; Col. 4:10)?
Answer: Yes, later it is assumed they were coworkers again.

WHAT IS A COMMUNITY?

OBJECTIVES: By the end of the lesson participants will:
1. Define what a community is
2. List components of a community
3. Describe what a Christian community looks like.

INTRODUCTION
Read Acts 2:41-47 Scripture on how the believers formed a community after transformation. Then ask the SHOWD questions: What do you **see**? What was **happening**? Does this happen in **our** place? **Why** does it happen there? What can we **do** about it?

LESSON
I. What does a Community look like?
A. What is the size of this first major Christian community?
Answer: Adding to the 500+ believers (1 Cor. 15:6) plus Acts 2:41 of 3000 souls.

B. What did this community do? (vs. 42)
Answer: Were being taught, fellowship, breaking bread and prayer.

C. What other activity was this community doing? (vs. 43-47)
Answer: Observing wonders, had things in common, selling property and possessions, sharing, one mind, in temple, house to house, eating together, praising God, favor with people, Lord adding to their community daily.

D. Read Luke 5:1-11
Think back to Jesus starting his first small group.

E. How many were in this first group?
Answer: Three plus Jesus made up of Peter, James and John.

F. What did the first group do?
Answer: "Left everything and followed Jesus." (Luke 5:11).

G. Explain how Peter responds to Jesus initially in vs. 5-8.
Answer: Tells his story, showed respect, saw a miracle before their very eyes, got partners involved, knelt humbly in obedience.

H. How did the three men respond after seeing Jesus enter the situation? (vs. 9)
Answer: Everyone completely surprised at what happened. Go to John 21:3 as follow up.

II. Components of a Community
   A. What components make up a community? (Ask for examples and record on board)
Answer: Parts of a community: share interests, depend upon each other, similar background & experiences, same geographic area, follow same leadership (church, political, family), family ties, common customs (habits, beliefs, ceremonies), communication and language same, common economical resources, they **know** each other, and do things together.

   B. Do we need all these components to have a community? No, summarize what makes a community.
Answer: The more things in common the more a community. Common—unity.

   C. As a summary, develop a definition of community. Start and have group contribute as you make the definition on board.
Answer: Definition: A group of people, growing together, in same geographic area, sharing interests, work and identity that know each other and do things together.
Note: Webster dictionary states could be group of nations with common traditions, politics and economy.

III. Characteristics of a Christian Community

A. What is the Bible view of a Christian community? Break into groups of 3-5 people and have each group take two verses: Acts 2:42; Acts 4:32; Psalm 82:3; Matt. 25:35-36; 2 Cor. 3:18; Rom. 8:17; 2 Tim. 2:2-3; Matt. 7:12.

Acts 2:42: pray, communion, teach, fellowship

Acts 4:32: meet needs of each other.

Psalm 82.3: justice to poor and orphan, rights to afflicted and destitute.

Matt. 25:35-36: clothe naked, feed hungry, visit sick & prisoners.

2 Cor. 3:18: growing relationship with Jesus

Rom. 8:17: co-heirs with Jesus, share in His sufferings.

2 Tim. 2:2-3: entrust to faithful men who will teach others.

Matt. 7:12: Golden Rule—do unto others as you would have them do unto you.

B. How will the community change as more and more become Christians?

Answer: As people accept Jesus, the community will look more like the above Christian traits. PEOPLE WILL START TO REACH OUT.

BIBLICAL IMPORTANCE OF CHILDREN

OBJECTIVES: By the end of this lesson, participants will

1. Understand God's focus on children and determine why we should involve them in community activities.

2. Recognize and apply from Scripture how children were trained and provided good examples.

INTRODUCTION

Read story: We know a group of community workers who know every inch of the community in which they live, who are accepted by everyone, and who want to help their community, who will work hard (for short periods of time) and cheerfully (all the time). Last month the health worker used them to collect information about which children had been vaccinated in the village. Next Tuesday some of them will help to remind the community that the baby clinic is coming, and they will be at hand to play with the older children when mothers take their babies to see the nurse. Next month they plan to help the schoolteacher in a village clean-up campaign. Who are these workers?

Answer: These health workers are the boys and girls of the village and community.

Source: Aarons, A. Hawes, H and Gayton, J (1979), *CHILD-to-CHILD*, London: Macmillan.

LESSON
A. Why are children important in a community
Answers:

1. They are leaders of tomorrow.
2. They give life and vigor.
3. Because they can make people happy.
4. They work and contribute to family and community.
5. Their learning will last a long-time.
6. They can influence many people over a lifetime.

7. No old habits need to be corrected.

B. How do you think children are important to God?
Answers:
1. God loves them.
2. They are tender and can be taught.
3. They continue life in the community.
4. Children's minds are moldable, open, and eager to learn and do.
5. Special because they are vulnerable.
6. They are defenseless.
7. Fresh from the Creator's hands.

C. Why are children important in the following Bible references?
Answers:
1. Matthew 18:1-6 (Jesus loves them and likes their innocence.)
2. Matthew 18:6 (They believe Jesus.)
3. Matthew 21:15-16 (They glorify God.)
4. 2 Timothy 3:15 (They understand Scriptures.)
5. Mark 10:13-16 (They come to Christ.)
6. Acts 2:39 (They receive the promises.)
7. Ephesians 6:4 (They receive training.)
8. 1 Samuel 1:24, 28 (They worship in God's house.)

D. What duties does the Bible say children have?
Answers:
1. Ephesians 6:1-4 (To obey parents who are following the Lord, to honor parents and care for them. They should follow discipline and instruction of the Lord.)
2. Hebrews 12:9 (Earthly fathers do discipline; children should respect their fathers.)

E. How should children be trained?
Answers:
1. Proverbs 22:6 (Children should be trained in his bent or God given direction or interests and talents.)
2. Deuteronomy 6:7 (They should be taught from the heart,

talk of God's word while sitting in home, when you walk by the way, when you lie down, and when you rise up.)

F. Give some examples of good children and why you think they are good.
Answers: Good children show love, respect, eagerness, and kindness. They want to please, benefit and improve the family, be contributing part of the family, dependable with jobs, do not complain, does what is asked to do.

G. Give examples of good children in the Bible.
Answers:
　　1. Genesis 22:6-10—Isaac (Trusting and faithful, willing to work.)
　　2. Genesis 45:9, 10—Joseph (Helps and wants best for family.)
　　3. 1 Samuel 2:26—Samuel (He grew in stature, favor with God and favor with men.)
　　4. 1 Samuel 17:20—David (He eagerly gets to task, followed instruction of his father, sees that his responsibility is done. Trusted God with Goliath.)
　　5. Daniel 1:8—Daniel (He has resolved to do right, to follow God, respectfully asks permission, shows himself in humble manner under authority.)
　　6. Luke 1:80—John the Baptist (He grew, became strong spiritually, lived a humble life until God was to use him.)
　　7. Luke 2:51—Jesus (He was under authority to his parents.)
　　8. Matthew 21:15, 16—Jesus in Temple (When children praised God in the Temple, Jesus stood up for them because they praised God innocently even though it was against what adults and leaders thought should be done.)
　　9. 2 Timothy 3:15—Timothy (He learned God's word from a very young age.)

H. How can children help to make your community a better place for everyone?
Answers:
　　1. Obey parents and Godly adults.

2. Learn Scriptures at early age.

3. They can lead other children in how to praise God.

4. When decisions have to be made, they can decide to do what God wants.

5. When given responsibility they should do the tasks well as unto the Lord.

6. When given a job and taught how to do it, they will do it eagerly

I. What can you do to assist this to happen?
Answers:

1. Help in family, church and community to encourage participation by children.

2. Show children the benefits of being healthy in learning, good relationships and a clean environment.

3. Encourage children to stay healthy and practice healthy habits.

4. Improve neighborhood environment by clean-up campaigns.

5. Pass their knowledge and skills to those who do not have it.

6. Help the needy and poor you know.

WHAT IS GOOD HEALTH?
[Adapted from Community Health Evangelism]

OBJECTIVES: By the end of this lesson, participants will:

1. Understand that God made everything healthy, but sin adversely affected our health.

2. Describe good health as living in harmony and being whole.

INTRODUCTION
Read Luke 5:17-26 about the healing of the paralytic. Then ask the SHOWD questions: What do you **see**? What was **happening**? Does this happen in **our** place? **Why** does it happen (or NOT happen) there? What can we **do** about it?

LESSON
A. What are the essentials for a person to live a healthy life? [Discuss in large group.]
Answer: Water, food, shelter, air, social encouragement, knowledge of life, mental understanding, etc.

B.   God created everything, and it was good. What does Genesis say about this?
   1. **What does Genesis 1:1 tell us about God & creation?**
Answer: *"In the beginning God created the heavens and the earth."* God is separate from creation.
   2. **What does Genesis 1:10, 12, 18, 21, 25 say about God and creation?**
Answer: God created water, plants, light, sea animals, beasts of the earth, and all is good.
   3. **In vs 26-27, what did God also make on the 6th day? In what image?**
Answer: Man, *"God created man in His own image, in the image of God He created him…"* God created people for a relationship with

117

them. Relationships were perfect, like God is perfect. Harmony and peace were with themselves, others, and all other creation (nature).

C. What happened with this harmony, completeness, and wholeness in Genesis chapter 3?
Answer: Relationships were broken when the sin of disobedience was done by Adams and Eve.

Good Health Defined and Described
A. The bible uses the word "shalom" to describe peace with God. We have peace with God when we have harmony and completeness in all our relationships. What is good health?
Answer: When we have peace, wholeness, well-being, and harmony between all our relationships—between God and self, God and others, God and nature.

B. What does it look like to live with harmony in all our relationships? [Break into groups with each group assigned and then discussing a different relationship and what harmony would look like in it.]
 1. **Harmony with Self**
 2. **Harmony with Others**
 3. **Harmony with Nature**
 4. **Harmony with God**
Answer:
 1. Self: Happy, peace, relationship with God, good health in physical, spiritual, mental and socially, understand sin affects on us and need to resolve with God, when disease comes rest in God.
 2. Others: Share with others, love our neighbor as ourselves, we should love other people, help others, be at peace with self, be aware others can give us disease and we can give them diseases.
 3. Nature: All earth and creation around us was made by God: wind, rain, etc. are part of natural creation, small organisms like bacteria and germs can affect us, to be in harmony we must live with all our surroundings, do not destroy what God has made, respect His land and animals.

4. God: Build a relationship with Jesus, get to know God through the Bible, pray to God regularly, live in righteousness, seek His will and obey it, praise Him & give Him glory, trust Him like a child would do, accept what God provides, study His word (bible), look to Him for our needs.

C. What is illness?
Answer: Disharmony in any one of the four areas of a person's life.

D. What is healing
Answer: Restoring harmony in any of the areas where there has been disharmony.

E. What do we need in each of the four relationships to have excellent health?
Answer:
1. Self—stability, self-esteem, self-acceptance, intimacy, purpose, value ourselves, humility
2. Others—relationships, love others, acceptance of others, safety, fit in society, freedom
3. Nature—clean air & water, education on creation, shelter, good food, medical care, exercise
4. God—relationship with God, obey & grow closer with Him, stewardship, discipleship

Our Personal Health
A. Read Luke 2:52 and 1 Samuel 2:26. What parts of a person are growing in each story?
Answer: mental, physical, spiritual, and social.

B. Think of the paralytic you read about in Luke 5:17-26. What parts of him became whole and complete?
Answer: mental (vs. 26), physical (vs. 23), spiritual (vs.20), and social (vs. 18-19).

C. Explain what happened in each of these four parts to show the paralytic and his friends growing & healing.

Answer:

Mental (26): Everyone saw and learned about the power of God.

Physical (24-25): A paralytic was able to rise up and walk.

Spiritual (20): Faith of paralytic and his friends bring forgiveness of sins.

Social (18-19): Men helping a paralytic friend who was in need.

DISCUSSION GUIDE

"Come now, and let us reason together," Says the Lord...
Isaiah 1:18a
*Study to shew thyself approved unto God, a workman that needeth
not to be ashamed, rightly dividing the word of truth.*
2 Timothy 2:15 (KJV)

Introduction

The church reaching out to communities, both local and international, is surely what Jesus had in mind when he proclaimed the Great Commission (Matthew 28:18-20). The Great Commission is the message of the resurrected Jesus to his disciples — *go therefore and make disciples of all nations*...It includes people across the street and people on the other side of the world. People are going beyond their church's walls and entering communities that need Christian development.

A key issue facing the church today is a strategy on how to go to these communities, neighborhoods, schools, regions, or countries; then what to do when you get there. *Step Outside of Your Church, Expand Your World* has attempted to assist you in working through these issues by setting a framework for you to make plans. This Discussion Guide is organized using the major headings of each chapter followed by a series of discussion questions. The questions are designed to stimulate your thinking and discussion on how to enter and lead in your community of choice.

Proceed through this Discussion Guide at your own pace as an individual or in a group. By reading *Step Outside of Your Church, Expand Your World,* the desire is not for you to get entangled in detail, but to encourage you to think how you, your group, or church can plan community outreach. Ideas have been given in the reading, but each community is different, therefore each community needs unique individual plans. The hope is for you to apply the ideas and principles in your area of influence and opportunity. As your group advances through these discussion questions, it will prove very helpful to have a recorder or secretary keep a notebook of answers for future reference.

The ultimate objective of this Discussion Guide is implementation of principles that will lead to a partnership with a community. If you are thinking about what a community is, you might consider how Webster defines community: "a group of people forming a smaller social unit within a larger one, and sharing common interests, work, identity, location, etc." An additional definition in Webster is, "a group of nations loosely or closely associated because of common traditions or for political or economic advantage" (*Webster's New World College Dictionary*, 2002). A community can be a few people in a group or a number of nations who have common unity together. That partnership will lead to a changed community that will increasingly practice and follow the Lord Jesus Christ.

Discussion Questions

1—REACHING OUTSIDE OF YOUR CHURCH
My Story (Page 13)

1.1 In the first sentence, Rabe says, stepping outside of your church to minister in a community will give you a new vision. Do you agree? Why or why not?

1.2 Have you ever asked Jesus into your life in prayer? Describe that transformation. What was your next step?

1.3 How did that next step include an initial group or community?

1.4 Looking back, what communities have you had influence with since your transformation? Explain how that influence looks.

A Big Step Outside My Church Ministry (Page 15)

1.5 Explain how you think a friend, ambassador, and servant are similar and different.

Going Through the Periods of Development (Page 16)

1.6 After being transformed by Jesus, what specific awareness or example should you have showing the needs of another person or group of people? From the seven Periods of Development, identify what period you are currently in. Why do you think this? Give examples.

1.7   What is currently happening in your life that encourages you to go to the next Period of Development? What do you expect will happen? How will that look?

1.8   As your time being a Christian increases, you will have many more experiences. Dream ahead as to what you would consider to be ideal. In 10 years? In 30 years? In 50 years?

A Biblical Example of Development (Page 21)

1.9   Just knowing some of the life of Jesus, what makes Him so life-like, a person you could sit with along the beach and discuss ideas of your life?

1.10 Why do you think the Antioch church was where believers were first called Christians?

1.11 If you were Barnabas, would you seek after Saul so you could teach together in a community that needed to learn about God? Why or why not?

1.12 What kind of character, attitude, and behavior do you think Barnabas had that caused him to be so successful with the disciples in Jerusalem, with Saul and those in Antioch?

1.13 When Paul did the leading, especially with Elymas the magician/sorcerer, how do you think Barnabas responded and felt?

1.14 Paul and Barnabas had a "sharp dispute" over a major doctrinal issue in Acts 15. Could they have avoided that? How or why not?

Outline of a Strategy (Page 23)

1.15 We know community development can be with a person, a church, a region, a country, or beyond. Why would you want to start small within your own area of influence?

1.16 In beginning community development, why is it important to develop close relationships with a person who is like-minded?

1.17 When you are meeting with your group of a few Christian people, why should you focus on a systematic planned study of the Bible or a Christian book as opposed to studying any topic of interest?

1.18 What New Testament Biblical examples do you find that show people making outreach to communities? See Jesus in Matt. 4:23, 9:35; John the Baptist in Matt. 3:5-6; Centurion in Matt. 8:5-13; and Paul in Acts 26.

1.19 When we see a group of people in a community where God is drawing our attention, an opportunity where people have needs, most of us desire to assist. Why is that true?

1.20 Each of us sees people with needs through our own interests, education, perspective or lens. Why must we be careful in planning specific community development action with people in the community we are partnering with for service? Are we biased?

1.21 When we partner with a community to do an outreach service, why is it so helpful to have a Community Committee of Insiders?

1.22 Think through your exit strategy. How and when should exiting be shared with the insiders? What good reasons exist for outsiders to become independent of insiders? Why is use of local resources so important?

The Future (Page 28)

1.23 How should relationships in the previous community change when you move on to work in another community?

1.24 What is the relational difference in a community between being a friend, ambassador, or servant?

1.25 Do you agree that we have two alternatives: selfishness or sacrifice? Why or why not?

2—GOING BEYOND THE ORDINARY

Background (Page 31)

2.1 How do you feel when you travel out of your community, especially into a community that is much different than you are accustomed to?

2.2 What would encourage you to commit to going to another community to share Jesus Christ?

Follow-up to a Dream (Page 32)

2.3   Consider a dream or vision you would like to achieve. Try to share that with close friends and see if they can understand it. What do you need to do to gain their understanding?

2.4   Share an experience you have had doing a group project. How did that experience change people's lives who are *inside* the group and *outside* the group?

What then is included in International Health?   (Page 33)

2.5   Think of your personal health—what comes to your mind when you think of community health?

2.6   Rabe outlines three problems with the WHO definition of health. Do you agree or disagree? Explain. What difference does it make?

2.7   What good reasons exist in your mind for physical and spiritual health to be reviewed and developed together? Explain what Rowland and also Moffitt think about this.

2.8   Moffitt states, "Biblical development reflects God's mind for man, while secular development's goals are developed from man's mind." What is the meaning of this statement? What different outcomes would you expect from each of these ideas?

A Basis for International Development Transformation (Page 35)

2.9   In Chapter 2 it states, "International health provides a broad basis for international development." What connections do you see between international health and international development?

2.10 After reading the material on Christian transformation, explain it in your own words and state why it is so important.

2.11 If behaviors and consequences develop out of beliefs and values, where should you focus your attempt to assist community participants to change their behavior? Give examples.

2.12 Why should you approach communities with an attitude of learning? How does this build relationships?

2.13 God has set four (Elliston states three) key relationships essential for the development worker who enters a community. How do you build harmony in each of these relationships?

Christian International Development encompasses Transformational Distinctives (Page 38)

2.14 Cite four Essential Distinctives and explain how you have used or observed each in practice.

2.15 Cite four Additional Distinctives and state why you would or would not use each.

Concluding Remarks (Page 42)

2.16 Explain what Rabe is asking for when he states, "It is about God and who He is!"

2.17 What does Rabe mean when he states, "What we do need is a bigger picture of God and He will give us a bigger picture of transformation?"

3—BUILDING PARTNERSHIPS
Background of a Problem (Page 45)

3.1 What is the relationship between capacity building of local participants as it relates to the sustainability of teaching and project work in that community?

3.2 In your own words, define capacity building.

3.3 Why do you think public private partnerships (PPPs) are essential for successful community development with people and programs?

3.4 In your selected community, cite the partners/stakeholders, services they could provide, and three outcomes you would expect.

3.5 Why do you think capacity building in NGOs and churches is not common?

3.6. What are the reasons for building greater relationships with participants in the community where we are advocating development?

3.7 Over time working together, why should outsiders decrease in their influence and insiders increase in influence?

3.8 What would an exit strategy look like in a community where you would like to work? How would you implement that exit strategy?

Transformational Development in Capacity Building (Page 50)

3.9   What does it mean that transformation needs to take place in participants within the community you want to change?

3.10 Why is the spiritual component so important in transformation of community participants?

3.11 In your own words, define transformational development.

3.12 Why is it so important that the initial training of community participants includes spiritual integration? Explain.

Distinctives for Successful Christian International Development (Page 53)

3.13 Even though many of the distinctives are common sense, why do you think it is so important to keep referring to them and discussing them?

3.14 Of the ten Essential Distinctives, select four and cite how you would use them.

3.15 Select four Additional Distinctives and explain the background of the Bible verses cited. Explain how the Bible verse supports the distinctive.

Key Distinctives for Capacity Building (Page 57)
Holistic ministry is taught

3.16 In the "Holistic ministry is taught" distinctive, why is human sin so important to consider?

3.17 What does Rabe mean when he states, "That result [separating physical and spiritual] is a split Christian mind followed by a separated behavior?"

3.18 Read 2 Corinthians 10:5 and Colossians 1:18. How do these relate to holistic ministry?

Community ownership is established

3.19 In reading Acts 2:44, we see believers take community ownership. Why is it important to have some believers in leadership?

3.20 Why is it essential for sustainability to have local people empowered?

Participatory methods of teaching are used

3.21 What key principles can you learn from this statement? "There is a major difference between the teacher telling as contrasted with the student learning" as you work with community people.

3.22 Why would the best learning take place when participants are involved?

3.23 Review a few CHE lessons online and identify characteristics of participatory learning in those lessons.

Community provides local resources for use in projects

3.24 Explain why, to be sustainable, answers to needs must come from within the community.

3.25 Why would a sense of good pride come when local resources are used?

Community committee is responsible with outside consultation

3.26 Why do you think the Scriptures (e.g. Prov. 11:14) encourage many counselors or advisers to be involved in making community decisions?

3.27 What do you think a community committee should do if they just cannot resolve an issue?

Conclusion (Page 61)

3.28 Explain and give reasons why outsiders building a relationship with community people is as important as outsiders bringing technical skills into the community?

4—GROWING STEP BY STEP

Introduction (Page 63)

4.1 Compare and contrast what development broadly means to people.

4.2 How is transformational development different from or like what you believe?

What is Development? (Pages 63)

4.3 What are the major differences between people-centered development and economic development?

4.4 Would you agree with Korten that the spirit component of development should be defined by the community in which you are working? Why or why not?

4.5 The "web of lies" in which the poor are caught can be very overpowering if it is allowed. Cite two examples and explain why they are lies. Explain the truth about each?

4.6 From a Christian perspective, why would you say sin is the cause of poverty?

4.7. Give examples in each dimension—mental, physical, spiritual, social—as to how people can be relieved from poverty through development.

4.8 From the CHE strategy, what positive principles would you encourage?

Why then Development? (Page 66)

4.9 When working with people and communities, why is having a Christian perspective, being transformed, so important?

4.10 How and why will a community usually take on the perception of the development worker leading the program? Explain.

Background—A Development Agency Case Study (Page 67)

4.11 Food for the Hungry (FH) is a Christian relief and development organization Rabe worked in as the Health Officer for ten years. Their mission statement logo was "meeting physical and spiritual needs worldwide." Based upon the little you know of Rabe's background, what do you think he did?

4.12 The FH organization began with the same vision that most development workers have in their first development experience. What stimulates such agencies and people?

4.13 Why do organizations and people eventually transition from relief to development?

4.14 What are the positives and negatives of a relief and development organization having most of their staff members working in countries of their birth?

4.15 Give three examples of relief and three examples of development. Explain what these might look like in a community you are familiar with.

4.16 Why do you think Vision of Community is so important?

Characteristic Periods of Development in Agency and Personnel (Page 69)

4.17 When an agency or staff starts reacting to organizational changes rather than being pro-active in change, what do you think is happening? What is the problem and how should it be solved?

4.18 As a potential development worker/missionary/disciple maker, what period are you in? Why do you think you are in this period?

4.19 What plans are you making to advance to the next period?

Progressive Characteristics of Development Work in Mission (Page 76)

4.20 Of the ten Essential Distinctives, select four and describe how you could apply each distinctive. Give real-life examples.

4.21 Select four Additional Distinctives and explain the background of the Bible verses cited. Describe how applying the Bible verses can help in your life and ministry.

Concluding Remarks (Page 79)

4.22 As organizations and personnel proceed through the seven characteristic Periods of Development, why would they also mature in their spiritual journey?

4.23 Explain why you can be in any of the seven development periods and still be in God's will?

4.24 Read Ephesians 5:25-27 for a big picture of God. What did Christ do for the church? What does it look like if you do the same for those you influence?

5—GIVING GENEROUSLY
Introduction (Page 81)

5.1 Read Luke 10:25-37, The Good Samaritan story. Of the six people shown in the story, which are you most like? Explain why.

5.2 When confronted with people who have needs, what is your usual response?

5.3 Describe a circumstance you have been in where you were confronted by a needy person. Share your response. How would you change your response?

5.4 Who would you say your neighbor is? How should you respond to him/her? Explain.

5.5 Describe the difference between being an insider as compared to being an outsider. Give characteristics of both.

Definitions (Page 83)

5.6 Why is development, defined as transformational development, so key to the Christian vision for development?

5.7 In the definition of Development Aid, what are the positive characteristics you see that are important?

Goals of Development and Humanitarian Assistance (Page 84)

5.8 Consider the reasons that aid and assistance may be given, then select two good reasons and two poor reasons. Explain why each would be good or poor.

5.9 Of the goals that should be worked towards for development and humanitarian assistance, what do you think advocating, bringing, and providing should look like?

5.10 From a major agency like the Red Cross, we see Community Restoration and Rebuilding, along with Disaster Preparedness, as key areas of involvement for development. How can you be involved with these in community development?

5.11 Do you think government and other agencies are taking community development ministries away from the church? Why or why not? What is the outcome?

5.12 How do The Great Commandment and The Great Commission demonstrate the goals of the church for community development?

Biblical Standards for Giving Aid (Page 88)
Attitude of the Giver Must Be True (Page 88)
5.13 Can a giver have and show a true heart, a generous commitment, and be cheerful, all at the same time? Review the Bible verses stated in numbers 1, 2, 3. Explain and give examples.

5.14 Per #4 principle, "Personal investment is made." Share how that would look in your life.

5.15 In #8 principle, "Giving to get something in return is not acceptable." Read the bible verse and explain why and how this is a major issue today. Give examples.

True Sacrifice is Giving Something of Value (Pages 91)

5.16 Read 1 Chron. 21:22-24 and explain why David would insist upon paying the full amount for the threshing floor land that Araunah wanted to give to him.

5.17 What cost did the disciples pay for following Jesus? Cost for the rich young ruler (Matt. 19:21-22)? Cost for you?

Give Proportional to What You Have Been Given (Page 92)

5.18 In #2, why would God want us to give to God first and give our best? Is this a test?

5.19 In #5, what does it mean to give sacrificially?

General Scriptural Principles of Giving (Page 94)

5.20 How does giving liberally to the needy set an example?

5.21 Why is showing compassion and getting involved in people's lives so important?

Problems with Humanitarian Aid and Development Assistance (Page 95)

5.22 Perhaps the greatest problem with giving humanitarian aid is that those receiving the aid (insiders) will become dependent on those giving the aid (outsiders). How can effectiveness, politics, economy, and social side effects be harmed when aid is given? Give examples.

5.23 Problems with humanitarian aid can be numerous. Select three of the ten mentioned at the end of the chapter (e.g. Efficiency and Effectiveness) and give examples. Then explain how these problems can be avoided.

Conclusions & Recommendations (Page 97)

5.24 There are many ways we can improve humanitarian aid. Select three of the eight. Give examples and explain.

5.25 Review #5 and #7 and explain the ideas and then give practical examples that could be used in real life to improve giving of aid.

EPILOGUE

Commentary (Page 99)

1. Why do you think John, the writer of Revelation, ends the last words in the Bible with, *"The grace of the Lord Jesus be with all. Amen"* (Revelation 22:21). Was this a final warning?

2. What do you think Jesus is demonstrating and saying when He establishes the church at Caesarea Philippi, especially with the poor reputation and sinfulness of the region?

Interpretation (Page 101)

1. How should the church be an organism rather than an organization?

2. How can local churches demonstrate Acts 1:8 in a thorough way?

An Example (Page 103)

1. How can students from China be an example of community development?

2. After reading the poem, describe the key principles of community development that are highlighted.

APPENDIX 1

Health Development Strategies
Training Schedule

Monday
Devotion: Great Commission/Commandment—Matt 25:35-40; 28:18-20; Luke 4:16-21; Is. 61:1-2
- A. Introduction Techniques & Expectations
- B. Health Development Strategy Core
- C. Define Vision of Community & Why
- D. How to Overcome Obstacles

Tuesday
Devotion: Integration of Physical and Spiritual—Luke 10:27
- A. What is Community and What is Development?
- B. Introduction to FHI Child Dev. Program Health Strategies booklet or Biblical Importance of Children
- C. What is Good Health—Luke 2:52
- D. What is Evangelism and Why Evangelize

Wednesday
Devotion: Paralytic in Luke 5:17-26
- A. Needs and Resources from God's Perspective
- B. Community Committee Role
- C. Motivating a Change in Behavior
- D. Importance of Follow-up

Thursday
Devotion: Barnabas—Acts 9:10-31; 11:19-28; 12:25-13:12
- A. How Jesus Taught—Matt. 10
- B. LePSAS Learning Technique
- C. Developing a Lesson Plan (Knowledge, Reflection, Decision, Action)
- D. Practice or Visit to Demonstration Project

Friday

Devotion: Our God is Sovereign--Job 42; Psalm 145:8-13
   A.   The Community Exit Strategy
   B.   Action Plans for Future Focus
   C.   Share & Pray
   D.   Final Questions, Evaluations and Close

APPENDIX 2

Health Development Strategy in Guatemala

MISSION: To inspire communities in Guatemala to healthy living through education, practice of positive skills and service to those in need.

MISSION LOGO: Meeting physical and spiritual needs in Guatemala

VISION: To see marginalized and disadvantaged people in Guatemala living healthy lives.

CORE VALUES:
- Collaboration, cooperation and coordination are essential to achieving our ENDS.
- Sustainability is a goal to be integrated into all planning realizing that self-sustainability of projects may require much patience and many years.
- True partnership is required for success. Local ideas and input must be given the highest priority in the planning process. True partnership involves a health inter-dependency that works to maintain a sense of equality between all members.
- Health Development Guatemala values the sharing of resources and ideas.
- All humans are of equal value and as such we serve the needs of the poor in Guatemala regardless of race, gender or religious affiliation.
- We value engaging the world on issues of health and community development. This allows for more opportunities to share the good news of Jesus Christ and His sacrifice on the cross.
- Accountability and transparency are essential.
- We value the power of prayer.

- We adhere to the Lausanne Covenant.
- We believe all should have access to good basic health services.

ENDS & OUTCOMES for which we strive:
- Those whom we serve will understand the biblical concept of "health."
- Synergy will be achieved creating cooperation, coordination and collaboration between governmental agencies and those NGO's, charitable organizations and other entities interested in seeing the poor in Guatemala have access to good basic holistic health services.
- Those who seek to engage in short term health related mission work will do so with a view towards long term results.
- A balance will be achieved between improving health systems capacity and community health development.
- The local church will be strengthened because of our work.
- Health Development Guatemala will be a learning organization.
- Health Development Guatemala will see to avoid creating or adding to the problem of dependency in Guatemala.
- Individual lives will be transformed and will transform their own communities and cultures.
- Health Development Guatemala will see to avoid creating or adding to the problem of dependency in Guatemala.
- Individual lives will be transformed and will transform their own communities and cultures.

APPENDIX 3

Health Development Strategies
Lesson Options

1. Devotions
   A. God is Sovereign—Job 42; Ps. 145:8-13
   B. Great Commission/Great Commandment
   C. Paralytic
   D. Barnabas
   E. Spiritual Warfare
   F. Integration of Physical and Spiritual
   G. Biblical Importance of Children
   H. Self-Evaluation of Jesus—John 17
   I. Unity in Teamwork
   J. Standing Strong: Obeying God
   K. Others
   L. _____
   M. _____
2. Group Introduction Techniques
3. Vision of Community (Kingdom of God)
   A. Why VOC
   B. How to Overcome Obstacles
4. What is Good Health
5. HDS Core Principles
6. Needs & Resources
7. Training Team Role
8. Community Committee Role
9. Health Promoter Role
10. Goals & Objectives Writing
11. LePSAS method
12. Teaching Methods
13. How Jesus Taught
14. Writing a Lesson Plan

15. Starting a Health Program
16. Sharing the Gospel
    A. Evangelistic Picture Book
    B. Contextualization
17. Field Information Gathering
18. The Health Assessment
19. Stations in Health Assessment
20. Action Plans Development
21. How Adults Learn
22. Home Visits
23. Walking with Christ
24. The Bible and _____
25. The Bible and _____
26. Selecting Health Topics
27. Building Health Curriculum Topics
28. Teaching Resources
29. Using Teaching Resources
30. Health Topic Lessons
    A. General Nutrition
    B. Child Nutrition
    C. Breast Feeding
    D. Diarrhea
    E. Dehydration
    F. Worms
    G. Alcohol
    H. Other Drugs Abused
    I. Personal Hygiene
    J. Clean Water
    K. First Aid
       • Breathing & CPR
       • Bleeding
       • Wounds
       • Shock
       • Health & Cold
    L. Disease Prevention
    M. Other Health Lessons_____
    N. Other Health Lessons_____

O. HIV/AIDS
31. Introduction to Child-to-Child Teaching
    A. Child-to-Child Teaching Methods
    B. Evaluating Child -to-Child Teaching
    C. Lessons for Child-to-Child Teaching
    D. Lessons: Malaria, Nutrition for Eyes, AIDS, Safe Clean Water, Small Latrines, Hygiene, Handwashing, Worms.
32. Materials for Home Learning
33. Community Involvement
34. Health Promoter Reports
35. Introduction to Management
    A. Planning in Management
    B. Organizing Management
36. Writing Job Descriptions
37. Goals for Life
38. Introduction to Evaluation
39. Use of Teaching Aids
40. Working with the Church
41. Home Fellowships
42. Holistic Ministry
43. Others _____
44. Others _____
45. Others _____

REFERENCES

Ajulu, Deborah. 2001. *Holism in Development: An African Perspective on Empowering Communities*. Monrovia, CA: MARC Books, World Vision International.

Basch, Paul. 1999. *Textbook of International Health,* 2nd Ed. Oxford: Oxford University Press.

Barbolet, Adam. 2006. *Global Humanitarian Assistance*. London: Development Initiatives.

Beyond Intractability. www.beyondintractability.org and www. beyondintractability.org/essay/humanitarian_aid/

Blackaby, Henry and Blackaby, Richard and King, Claude, 2009. *Experiencing God*. Nashville: LifeWay Press.

Branczik, Amelia. 2004. *Humanitarian Aid and Development Assistance*. Boulder: University of Colorado.

Communitybuilders.nsw. 2001. URL: http://www.comunity builders.nsw.gov.au Progress Report: October 2001, "Management Support and Organizational Development" Working Group-16/10/01.

Cope, Landa L, a YWAM trainer. 2001. "Biblical Reflections—The Old Testament Template" paper presented at the Godmission.community 2001 AFMA/EFMA conference in Orlando, FL on September 21.

Chambers, Robert. 1997. *Whose Reality Counts? Putting First Last*. London: Intermediate Technology Publications.

Christian, Jayakumar. 1994. *Powerless of the Poor: Toward an Alternative Kingdom of God based Paradigm of Response*. Ph.D thesis at Pasadena, CA: Fuller Theological Seminary.

Easterly, William. 2006. *The White Man's Burden*. New York: The Penguin Press.

Elliston, Edgar J., Ed. 1989. *Christian Relief and Development*. Dallas: Word Publishing. Edited by Edgar Elliston.

Elliston, Edgar J. 1997. *Developing Leaders at a Distance Contextualizing Leadership Development.* Presented at ACCESS conference (January 15, 1998) Pasadena, CA: U.S. Center for World Mission.

Family Health International. 2002. "HIV/AIDS Prevention and Care Services." *Program Management and Support: Capacity Building,* January 26.

Firoz, Solmaz. 2005. *Human Rights Watch.* New York: Seven Stories Press.

Friedman, Thomas L. 2006. *The World is Flat.* New York: Farrar, Straus and Giroux.

Holman, Ben. 2002. "Change a Heart, Transform a Community." Scottsdale, AZ: *Newsletter of Food for the Hungry,* September.

Holy Bible. 1977. New American Standard Bible. La Habra, CA: The Lockman Foundation

Holy Bible. 1984. New International Version. Grand Rapids: Zondervan, International Bible Society.

International Institute for Environment and Development. URL: http://www.iied.org/resources for online database and URL: www.PLANOTES.ORG for journal notes. London, UK.

International Mission Board, IMB. See PeopleGroups.org-Lisu website.

Jayakaran, Ravi. 1996. *Participatory Learning and Action: User Guide and Manual.* Madras, India: World Vision India.

Johnstone, Patrick and Mandryk, Jason. 2001. *Operation World.* Waynesboro, GA: Paternoster Publishing.

Korten, David C. 1990. *Getting to the 21st Century: Voluntary Action and the Global Agenda.* West Harford, Conn: Kumarian Press.

Lisk, Franklyn. 1996. "Capacity Building for Management and Development." URL: http://euforic.org/courier. The Courier ACP-EU, No. 159, September-October.

Miller, Darrow L. 1998, 2001. *Discipling Nations: The Power of Truth to Transform Cultures.* Seattle, WA: YWAM Publishing.

Millham, Douglas E. 1989. *Training for Relief in Development in Christian Relief and Development.* Dallas: Word Publishing. Edited by Edgar Elliston.

Mission Frontiers. May-June 2004, Vol. 26, No. 3. Website: www.mission1.org. Pasadena, CA: The U.S. Center for World Mission.

Moffitt, Bob. 1995. *Distinctions of Biblical Development.* Tempe, AZ: The Harvest Foundation.

Myers, Bryant L. 1999. *Walking with the Poor: Principles and Practices of Transformational Development.* Maryknoll, NY: Orbis Books.

Myers, Bryant L. 1999. *Working with the Poor.* Maryknoll, NY: Orbis Books.

O'Donnell, K. 2002. *Doing Member Care Well: Perspective and Practices from around the World.* Pasadena, CA: William Carey Library.

Performance Management Solutions website. "Capacity building Through Management Development." URL: http://www.pm-solutions.com/Capacity_Building.html.

Rabe, Alan. 1993. *Be in Health*, 2nd. Ed. Dubuque, IA: Kendall/Hunt Publishing Company.

Rabe, Alan N. 2002. "Capacity Building for Management of Sustainable Holistic Development" in *The Journal of Management: International Development*, Vol. 1. Fullerton, CA: Hope International University. Edited by Raj Singh.

Rabe, Alan N. 2001. "Selected International Development Reflections for Transformational Distinctives." Unpublished paper presented at The Annual Dinner, Department of Management. Fullerton, CA: Hope International University. October 19.

Ram, Eric. 1995. *Transforming Health.* Monrovia, CA: MARC, World Vision International.

Reuter, Dieter. 2002. "Development Partnerships with the Private Sector and Global Training for Sustainable Development PPPs in Work of Carl Duisberg Gesellschaft (CDG)." *D+C Development and Cooperation*, No. 4, July/August.

Rowland, Stan. 1995. "Christian Witness through Community Health" in *Transforming Health*. Monrovia, CA: MARC Publications. Edited by Eric Ram.

Rowland, Stan. 2001. *Multiplying Light and Truth*. Mumbai, India: GLS Publishing.

Serving in Mission Together. Fall 2004, Issue 107. Website: www. hopeforAIDS.org. Charlotte, NC: Serving in Missions (SIM). Edited by Carol Wilson.

The American Heritage Dictionary, 2nd. Ed. 1982. Boston: Houghton Mifflin Company.

Vinay, Samuel and Sugden, Christopher, Eds. 1987. *The Church in Response to Human Need*. Grand Rapids: Eerdmans Publishing.

Webster's New World Dictionary, 4th Ed. 2002. Cleveland: Wiley Publishing, Inc.

Wheeler, Genevieve Elaine. November 2003. *Developing Effective Member Care Strategies within Food for the Hungry International*. Unpublished Master of Business Administration in International Development degree. Fullerton, CA: Hope International University.

Wikipedia. 2006. http://en.wikipedia.org/wiki/Humanitarian_aid. October 26.

World Health Organization. 1947. "Constitution of the World Health Organization" in *Chronicle of the World Health Organization*. New York: World Health Organization.

Yamamori, Tetsunao. 1993. *Penetrating Missions' Final Frontier*. Downers Grove, IL: InterVarsity Press.

ABOUT THE AUTHOR

Alan N. Rabe is currently retired, as much as a Christian should. He was founder of the Ministry Development Institute (MDI) at The Crossing church in Quincy, IL., Dean of School of Graduate Studies at Hope International University (Fullerton, CA.), Health Officer at Food for the Hungry International, and for some 30 years, taught public/community health at the State University of New York at Brockport, Central Michigan University, Illinois State University and Liberty University in Virginia.

Dr. Rabe is a graduate of Western Illinois University, the University of Illinois, and received a Ph.D. from the University of Utah. He completed the MRE degree from Liberty Baptist Theological Seminary. Alan is an ordained minister.

Currently, his major focus and passion is diverse. He reaches outside the church by teaching Bible in State prisons, serving as a chaplain in care facilities, and teaching pastors and church leaders in developing countries of the world. His personal mission is to dedicate himself to a personal relationship with Jesus Christ, try to follow Him, and influence others to serve those in need.

Alan and his wife Linda were high school sweethearts, have been married for over 50 years, and have two grown children. They make their home in Quincy, Illinois, near family farms where they both grew up.